ESSENTIAL

Ultrasound Anatomy

ESSENTIAL
Ultrasound Anatomy

Marios Loukas, MD, PhD
Dean of Basic Sciences and Research
Co-Chair Department of Anatomical Sciences
St. George's University
Grenada, West Indies

Danny Burns, MD, PhD
Department of Anatomical Sciences
St. George's University
Grenada, West Indies

Philadelphia • Baltimore • New York • London
Buenos Aires • Hong Kong • Sydney • Tokyo

Senior Acquisitions Editor: Crystal Taylor
Development Editor: Amy Millholen
Editorial Coordinator: Emily Buccieri
Editorial Assistant: Parisa Saranj
Marketing Manager: Tyrone Williams
Production Project Manager: Barton Dudlick
Design Coordinator: Elaine Kasmer
Manufacturing Coordinator: Margie Orzech
Prepress Vendor: TNQ Technologies

Throughout this book, a portion of the cadaveric images were made possible by using the NLM Visible Human Project®: http://www.nlm.nih.gov/research/visible/visible_human.html.

9 8 7 6 5 4 3 2 1

Printed in China

Library of Congress Cataloging-in-Publication Data

Names: Loukas, Marios, author. | Burns, Danny (Professor of anatomy), author.
Title: Essential ultrasound anatomy / Marios Loukas, Danny Burns.
Description: Philadelphia : Wolters Kluwer, [2020] | Includes index.
Identifiers: LCCN 2019003138 | ISBN 9781496383532
Subjects: | MESH: Ultrasonography–methods | Anatomy, Regional
Classification: LCC RC78.7.U4 | NLM WN 208 | DDC 616.07/543–dc23
LC record available at https://lccn.loc.gov/2019003138

shop.LWW.com

Dedications

To Marti, my spouse and best friend for her patience and support throughout the years. To my mentors in medical and graduate school, and to the many students and junior colleagues whose excitement about learning have made this journey so much fun. **–D.B**

To my daughter Nikol, my son Chris, and my wife Joanna for their patience and support putting up with my early mornings and late nights during the creation of this book. Love you so much. **–M.L**

Acknowledgments

We would like to thank all the donors and their families for their ultimate donation for the benefit of future generations of physicians and scientists. This book could have never materialized without their immeasurable contributions.

The production of the cadaveric materials is a huge team effort that has involved several faculty, laboratory technicians, and administrative staff.

We would also like to thank the following colleagues for their technical expertise in dissections and their enormous help with this project:

Rodon Marrast, Shiva Mathurin, Romeo Cox, Seikou Phillip, Marlon Joseph, Nelson Davis, Travis Joseph, Simone Francis, Charlon Charles, Arnelle Gibbs, Sheryce Fraser, Chad Phillip, Ryan Jacobs, Nadica Thomas-Dominique, Tracy Shabazz, and Yvonne James of the Department of Anatomical Sciences, St. George's University, School of Medicine, Grenada, West Indies, for their technical, laboratory, and administrative assistance.

The following faculty also assisted with this project:

Yusuf Oladimeji Alimi, Ms. Maira duPlessis, Seid Eid, Drs. Theofanis Kollias, Sasha Lake, Ahmed Mahgoub, Rabjot Rai, Ramesh Rao, Asad Rizvi, Wallisa Roberts, Sonja Salandi, and Deepak Sharma from the Department of Anatomical Sciences, St. George's University, School of Medicine, Grenada, West Indies.

Special thanks to Jennifer Kelly RDMS, RTNM, who was excited about this project from the very beginning and who spent countless hours obtaining many of the ultrasound images and videos used in this book and working with the St. George's University illustration team documenting patient positioning and probe placement.

We thank the following instructors of the Department of Anatomical Sciences, St. George's University, School of Medicine, Grenada, West Indies, for their contributions in illustrations: Jessica Holland, Brandon Holt, David Nahabedian, Luz Ortiz Nieto, Charles Price, Xochitl Vinaja, and Katie Yost. We are grateful for their hard work, talent, ideas, patience, and creativity and feel fortunate that they are our colleagues and friends.

Ultrasound allows physicians to see through the body in real time but necessitates significant training. Therefore, instructing future physicians at an early stage is important. Several years ago, we began teaching hands-on ultrasound anatomy to medical students in the basic sciences. We believe that the rapid pace of introduction of new clinical applications of ultrasound across nearly all specialties necessitates providing a solid foundation in ultrasound technique, anatomy, and physiology from the very beginning of medical education. The wide availability of point-of-care ultrasound imaging in clinics, emergency departments, and hospital wards has made ultrasound examination knowledge and skills in the 21st century every bit as critical as stethoscope examination knowledge and skills. From the beginning, one of the challenges was how to prepare students (as well as anatomy faculty) for hands-on sessions such that the time allotted for examining standardized patients was utilized to the best advantage. Early on, we recognized that too much laboratory time was spent explaining (and re-explaining) patient positioning and probe placement and the ultrasound appearance of local landmarks and key anatomical features. We wanted reference materials for students to prepare in advance and show up for laboratories with a basic understanding of optimal patient positioning for this or that ultrasound image, where to position the probe, and how to look for key landmarks and anatomical structures in real-time ultrasound images. In this way, laboratory sessions could begin and end with probes in students' hands, with instructors at their sides asking questions and providing guidance and suggestions as needed.

Most books and other resources for learning specific ultrasound techniques are aimed primarily at practitioners who are already utilizing ultrasound imaging in their clinical practice. Accordingly, much of the available information is focused on technical details of clinical applications. We hope this book provides a foundation in regional ultrasound anatomy, which is accessible to students from the very beginning of medical education and sufficiently detailed to be of interest to practitioners who are already incorporating ultrasound imaging into their daily practice. The book is organized by anatomical regions, and each section has a similar organization. Each section begins with an overview of the relevant anatomy ("Review of the Anatomy"), followed by a "Technique" section. Both sections describe in text and illustrate the important technical details and skills for obtaining specific ultrasound images from that region. Each figure includes the following components: an unlabeled ultrasound image, a labeled ultrasound image, and the same image "painted" with tissue texture such as muscle, tendons, organs (e.g., liver, kidney, muscle); a drawing demonstrating optimal patient positioning, probe placement, and probe indicator direction; and a labeled cadaver slice matching the ultrasound images. Each technique text section is tagged with a quick reference tab that identifies an ultrasound image orientation and content and references the specific figure where that image is found.

The book can be read by chapters/chapter sections "like a novel" as students encounter different anatomical regions in their coursework to get an overview of the kinds of ultrasound images and important structures that might be commonly encountered. Alternatively, individual ultrasound images from specific areas can be easily located along with illustrations and textual descriptions of how to obtain that image and identify structures and landmarks within the image. Course instructors could, for example, choose 2 or 3 images from an anatomical region and assign appropriate reading for student preparation for laboratory sessions in which students would be expected to appropriately position standardized patients, place probes in the correct location and orientation, and begin to navigate and identify landmarks and key structures from each of these images. A special chapter describing and illustrating normal and abnormal findings in the FAST examination has been introduced, giving readers an opportunity to apply ultrasound anatomy from the heart, upper quadrants of the abdomen, and male and female pelvis in the context of an important and commonly utilized clinical application of ultrasound. The final chapter contains several USMLE-type multiple-choice questions designed to provide feedback to students, instructors, and physicians in a clinically meaningful way.

We hope this book will provide everyone who is interested in exploring the use of ultrasound with a rational anatomical basis for locating and identifying important structures throughout the body.

Table of Contents

Table of Contents

1
Introduction

Ultrasound Basics

Ultrasound (US) is an imaging technology widely used across multiple medical specialties. The devices are portable and free of ionizing radiation, with low risk for harm even in the most vulnerable populations. The portability, safety, and relatively low cost of US imaging have made it widely available for bed-side and other point-of-care imaging, increasingly as an extension of the physical examination (e.g., examining the peritoneal spaces for the presence of free fluid when intraperitoneal bleeding is suspected) or for guiding interventional procedures, such as central line placement, nerve blocks, joint injections, and biopsies.

Typical US images display 2-dimensional slices of internal structures. Depending on the placement and orientation of the probe on the body surface, the image may be transverse, sagittal/parasagittal, coronal, or oblique. Images are acquired in real time, such that respiratory movements, ventricular contractions, arterial pulsations, phasic changes in venous blood flow, muscle/tendon/joint movements, or the effects of provocative stresses on

ligaments or tendons can all be easily observed by experienced operators.

From a transducer housed in the US probe, short pulses of very high frequency sound are transmitted across the body surface into the patient's body. As the US pulses propagate through the body and encounter tissues with different acoustic properties, some sound energy is reflected back to the transducer (echo) and some continues to penetrate to deeper tissues (through-transmission). The echo signals that return to the probe are processed and combined to generate an image of the slice being scanned.

Different Probes for Different Applications

IMAGE SHAPE AND DEPTH OF DIFFERENT PROBES FIG. 1.1

There are 3 commonly used surface probe types for most general-purpose US imaging applications: **abdominal probes**, **cardiac probes**, and **high-frequency linear probes**.

Linear   Curved array   Cardiac

cm
0

5

10

15

Figure 1.1 Linear, abdominal, and cardiac probes. The shape of the image produced by each probe type is depicted with blue shading.

Abdominal (Convex or Curved Array) Probes

These are low- to intermediate-frequency (2-5 MHz) probes with a curved face and a "footprint" of typically 4 to 6 cm (the side-to-side dimension of the probe face). As the name implies, these probes are commonly used for general purpose abdominal imaging, but they are also used for other applications such as transabdominal pelvic imaging, obstetrical imaging, and some musculoskeletal imaging, such as spine and hip joint. The relatively low frequencies available with these probes allow for imaging up to depths of 20 cm or so, and the sector image produced is the width of the probe footprint at the skin surface, becoming progressively wider as the depth increases. This allows for a wide-angle field of view for imaging large deeper structures (e.g., kidneys) and landmarks, but owing to the width of the footprint, it is also possible to image structures nearer the skin surface with a reasonably wide field of view.

Cardiac (Sector Array) Probes

These probes are used extensively in heart US imaging (echocardiography) but are well suited for imaging any relatively large, nonsuperficial structures through narrow sonographic windows (such as intercostal spaces). They produce a sector image that resembles a triangular shape, a very small (essentially a point source) surface footprint becoming progressively wider with increasing depth. The resonant frequency is low (1.5-4.5 MHz), allowing for substantial depth penetration (similar to abdominal probes). Because the image is so narrow at the surface, these probes are not useful for imaging superficial structures, but they can be adapted to most abdominal US imaging purposes if necessary.

Linear (Linear Array) Probes

Because of their high resonant frequencies (8-15 MHz) these probes offer the best image detail but poor depth penetration. Consequently, they are used for musculoskeletal, peripheral nerves, thyroid gland, breast, superficial vascular, and other imaging applications that require high-resolution images from relatively superficial tissues (approximately 5-6 cm maximum depth from the skin surface). The images they produce are rectangular in shape. The image width remains the same from the probe face at the surface to the deepest part of the image (the width of the probe footprint, commonly 4-5 cm).

Using Ultrasound Probes

Ultrasound Gel

The probe face must be coupled to the skin surface by using a water-based gel that has sound transmission

ULTRASOUND GEL ACOUSTICALLY COUPLES PROBES TO SKIN
FIG. 1.2

properties similar to skin. The gel also excludes air pockets between the probe face and the skin (or skin folds and irregularities), which would interfere with the transmission of US pulses into the skin and on to deeper tissues.

Controlling and Manipulating the Probe

To obtain quality images, US users must learn to control and manipulate the probe in terms of exerting an appropriate amount of pressure, stabilizing the probe face on uneven and slippery surfaces and making fine adjustments in the angle, rotation, and tilt of the probe face relative to structures of interest.

Most of the time, moderate, evenly applied pressure across the probe face is needed. The screen image drops out from areas of the probe face that does not make sufficient contact with the skin surface. Some US imaging tasks require greater pressures, whereas others need minimal pressures.

Proper rotation and tilting (**fanning** or **toggling**) of the probe face are critical to view structures of interest in their true longitudinal axis or transverse axis (and to change a view from longitudinal to transverse or vice versa) and to produce accurate images of structures that are not parallel to the skin surface. Some structures, including tendons and nerves, appear much brighter when the US beam is perpendicular to their course.

Because of probe pressure, probe movement across tender areas, and/or patient positioning, US scanning can occasionally be uncomfortable for patients, but it should never be unnecessarily uncomfortable or painful.

Gel

Skin

Air pocket

 Figure 1.2 Ultrasound gel acoustically couples the outermost layer of the probe face to skin.

Communicating with patients and paying careful attention to their comfort and safety is always a high priority during US scanning.

Probe and Display Orientation Markers

To understand the positions and relationships between structures in US images, you must be able to orient images in terms of superficial to deep and superior to inferior or left to right (lateral to medial). All US probes have an orientation marker on one side near the probe face, usually a raised dot or ridge along the side of the probe, and sometimes a small LED light. The probe orientation marker corresponds to an orientation marker on the display image, usually a colored dot or the manufacturer's logo. By convention, for most US imaging, the display orientation marker is placed on the upper left corner of the image. For historical reasons (not just to confuse medical students), the orientation marker is typically placed on the right side of the display for cardiac US. Also, by convention, the orientation marker on the probe should be directed superiorly (cephalad) when performing a scan along the long axis of the body and directed toward the right side of the patient when performing a scan that is transverse to the long axis of the body.

ORIENTING TO SCANS ACQUIRED ALONG THE LONGITUDINAL AXIS FIG. 1.3

When these conventions are followed, structures nearer the left side (marker side) of the image are more superior and structures nearer the right side (nonmarker side) of the image are more inferior in longitudinal scans. The image in Figure 1.3 was acquired along the longitudinal axis, with the probe face on the skin of the cubital fossa and the probe orientation marker directed superiorly. Knowing this, we can understand the orientation of the image and begin to identify structures and landmarks.

ORIENTING TO SCANS ACQUIRED ALONG THE TRANSVERSE AXIS FIG. 1.4

Similarly, following the conventions described earlier for transverse scans, structures on the marker side of the image are toward the patient's right and structures the nonmarker side of the image are toward the patient's left. The image in Figure 1.4 was acquired transverse to the longitudinal axis of the body (which is also transverse to the limb), with the probe face on the skin of the cubital fossa of the patient's right upper limb and the probe orientation marker directed to the right.

In all scans, structures nearer the top of the display image are more superficial and structures nearer the bottom of the image are deeper. The numbers and hash marks located along the side of the image indicate depth in centimeters.

QUICK TIP: Touching or tapping one edge of the probe face with your index finger while observing the screen image for a corresponding flicker is a quick and easy way to determine the probe orientation in relation to the display image.

Figure 1.3 Use of the probe marker and display marker to orient to images acquired in the longitudinal axis.

Appearance of Tissues in Ultrasound Images

ECHOGENICITY: GRAY-SCALE IMAGE DISPLAY
FIG. 1.5

Echogenicity refers to the amount of US reflection by a tissue relative to surrounding tissues. Whenever there is an interface between tissues with

APPEARANCE OF COMMONLY ENCOUNTERED TISSUES
FIG. 1.6

different echogenicities, a visible difference in brightness will be seen on the US display. Based on the degree of echogenicity, tissues or structures are described as hyperechoic (white on the display), hypoechoic (gray on the display), or anechoic (black on the display).

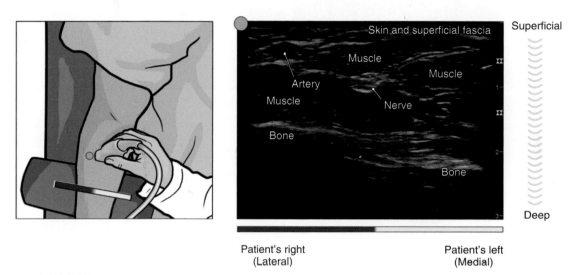

Figure 1.4 Use of the probe marker and display marker to orient to images acquired in the transverse axis.

Examples

Anechoic
Little or no echogenicity ="black" display
Fluids such as ascites, bile, urine, effusions, uclotted blood, fluid in cysts, subcutaneous fat

Hypoechoic
Low-intermediate echogenicity = "gray" display
Many tissues/organs such as skeletal muscle, spleen, liver, pancreas, kidney, uterus, myocardium

Hyperechoic
High echogenicity = "white" display
Pleura, pericardium, diaphragm, bone surfaces, tendons, ligaments, calcifications

Figure 1.5 Echogenicity and gray-scale image display.

Figure 1.6 Appearance of commonly encountered tissues in US images.

Skin

Skin appears smooth and bright (**hyperechoic**). The epidermis and dermis can be differentiated only with specialized high-resolution US. There is a very thin and bright epidermal entry echo followed by a slightly less hyperechoic band representing the epidermis and dermis. Immediately deep to the dermis, the subcutaneous fatty/fibrous layer appears generally hypoechoic (dark) in US images, with 2 components, **anechoic/hypoechoic** fat, interspersed with thin hyperechoic lines representing connective tissue septae.

Skeletal Muscle

Skeletal muscle has a distinct appearance, which varies between transverse views (across the long axis of the muscle) and longitudinal views (parallel to the muscle's long axis). In the transverse view, muscle tissue is largely anechoic-hypoechoic speckled with multiple short, thin, hyperechoic lines representing reflections from connective tissue of the perimysium. This is commonly referred to as the *starry sky* appearance.

In the longitudinal view, most of the muscle tissue remains anechoic/hypoechoic, but the hyperechoic lines of perimysium are elongated, revealing the fascicular architecture of the muscle. Most surfaces/boundaries of muscles are readily visible owing to the hyperechoic lines produced by the epimysium and the connective tissue of deep fascia.

Tendons

Tendons have a distinct appearance owing to the highly ordered, parallel bundles of collagen fibers that make up most of the tendon interior. As a result, multiple thin, hyperechoic lines fill in the tendon interior when viewed in the long axis of the tendon (commonly referred to as the *fibrillar* appearance) and there is a hyperechoic border (epitendineum investing the tendon) at the tendon surface.

In the transverse view, tendon interiors are filled in with many small, clustered, hyperechoic dots (commonly referred to as the *bristle-brush* appearance), again with a distinct hyperechoic surface (see Figure 1.6).

Nerves

Nerves have a largely hyperechoic surface and background (owing to reflectivity of connective tissue of the epineurium and perineurium) that is dotted with multiple hypoechoic nerve fascicles (the *honeycomb* appearance), when viewed in their transverse axis.

When viewed in the longitudinal axis, the nerve fascicles appear as multiple, thin, hypoechoic stripes parallel to the long axis of the nerve, against the hyperechoic background of the perineurium and surrounding epineurium (the *bundle of straws* appearance) (see Figure 1.6).

Bone

Bone surfaces appear as hyperechoic lines with a clean, dark, acoustic shadowing deep to the bone surface. For very small bony projections, acoustic shadowing is often the most obvious visual clue to their presence. Because bone surface is so reflective, artifacts (reverberations and *mirror images*) may appear within the acoustic shadow (see Figure 1.6).

Fluids

Fluids, such as blood, bile, and urine, are anechoic. In addition, sound energy propagates through fluid with minimal energy loss compared with soft tissues. This produces noticeably increased echogenicity in the tissues deep to fluid collections, because more sound energy reaches these tissues compared with the nonfluid sound path on either side of the fluid collection.

Blood Vessels

The blood (a fluid) flowing through the lumens of arteries and veins is anechoic (unless clots are present), whereas the connective tissue in vessel walls is hyperechoic. Arteries tend to have a more circular profile in transverse view than veins (which tend to be more oval), and artery walls are thicker than comparably sized veins (see Figure 1.6). Arterial and venous pulsations can be easily seen in real-time images (this can be confusing at times). However, normal veins are readily compressible by exerting minimal pressure on the probe, whereas arteries are only compressed with substantial pressure.

Basic "Knobology" and Image Optimization

During every US examination, US machine settings should be changed *as needed* to optimize image quality. Understanding what just a few of the machine's knobs do is sufficient for optimizing most routine scans.

Depth

SCAN DEPTH AND FOCAL POINT INDICATORS
FIG. 1.7

The scan depth is indicated in centimeters on the right side of the image. In general, it is a good idea to start with greater depth to visualize more structures and landmarks in the field in addition to the structure/region of interest. After orienting yourself to the structures in the image and identifying the region of interest, readjust the depth so that the region of interest is located near the center of the display.

Muscle (oblique view)

Muscle (longitudinal view)

Artery

Nerve (transverse view)

Vein

Focal depth marker

Depth scale

Figure 1.7 Scan depth and focal depth markers.

Focal Points

Most contemporary US units allow the user to set one or more focal depths. Focal depths are indicated alongside the depth markers. For example, the image in Figure 1.7 shows a scan depth of 4 cm, and there are 2 focal points selected (the yellow *hourglass* icons), set at 1.0 cm and at 2.25 cm.

In general, 2 or 3 focal points should be chosen and distributed near the depth(s) that correspond to the region of interest. This will provide the best image detail for structures near the focal depth(s).

Gain

Turning the gain knob increases or decreases the amount of amplification of echoes throughout the image, increasing or decreasing the overall brightness of the displayed image. Images that are neither too bright nor too dark are best for overall identification of structures (inexperienced examiners tend to choose too much gain).

Tissue Harmonics Imaging

US pulses are produced in the probe transducer at some fundamental frequency (e.g., 12 MHz for a typical high-frequency linear array transducer). As the pulse travels through tissues, the tissues themselves vibrate at multiples of the fundamental frequency (2X = first harmonic, 4X = second harmonic, etc.). The tissue harmonics button on the US device toggles between listening for echoes at the fundamental frequency and listening for echoes only at harmonic frequencies. Tissue harmonics imaging frequently results in improved image quality, in terms of decreases in some artifacts (reverberations), decreased noise throughout the image, fewer internal echoes in fluid-filled spaces (cyst clearing), and improved image detail (spatial resolution).

2

Basic Ultrasound Physics

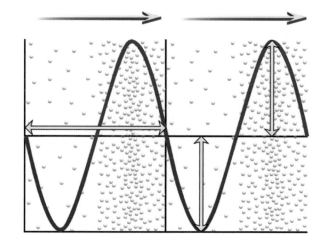

Sound Waves

SOUND WAVE PROPAGATION FIG. 2.1

Sound is a mechanical wave of alternating pressures that propagates through media (such as tissues) as a series of compressions as the wave pressure rises and rarefactions as the wave pressure falls of the molecules in the medium. Sound cannot travel through a vacuum.

Sound can be characterized by many different parameters, but one important characteristic of sound is its frequency (number of cycles per unit time, most commonly cycles per second, or Hertz).

One cycle per second = one Hertz (Hz)
One thousand cycles per second = one kilohertz (KHz)
One million cycles per second = one megahertz (MHz)

Therefore, a 12-MHz transducer in a medical ultrasound (US) probe (a "12-MHz probe") transmits pulses with a fundamental frequency of 12,000,000 cycles per second.

Another feature of sound is its velocity. Sound velocity in a given material is constant (at constant temperature), but velocity varies in different materials. Sound velocity through most soft tissues is fairly similar, although there are some extremes such as lungs (600 m/s) and dense bone (4000 m/s). For image forming, US devices assume that the velocity of sound through tissues is 1540 m/s, the soft tissue average.

US PULSE: REFLECTION AND THROUGH-TRANSMISSION FIG. 2.2

FORMING AN IMAGE: REFLECTION (ECHO) AND THROUGH-TRANSMISSION FIG. 2.3

In US image forming, an important characteristic of the media (tissues) through which sound energy propagates is **acoustic impedence**, the product of sound velocity through a tissue and the tissue density. Most soft tissues have similar acoustic impedence values, but there are some extremes such as bone, lungs, and collections of air/gas (e.g., alveolar air, bowel gas). When sound passes from one tissue (with some value of acoustic impedance) to another tissue (with a different acoustic impedance), some of the sound is reflected at the interface between the 2 tissues and some continues on to be transmitted to deeper layers—the greater the difference in impedance the greater the amount of sound reflection.

Because the impedance values are similar for most tissues, only a small amount of the sound pulse energy is reflected at tissue interfaces. This acoustic matching is good for imaging purposes, as a small amount of energy is reflected back to the probe as echoes for image forming, whereas most of the energy is transmitted on deeper to the next interface to be reflected to form an image there, and so on through the depth of the area being scanned (see Figure 2.3).

BARRIERS TO US IMAGING: BONE AND AIR FIG. 2.4

By the same logic, imaging problems arise when US pulses encounter an interface between tissues with large differences in acoustic impedance, such as soft tissue to bone or soft tissue to air.

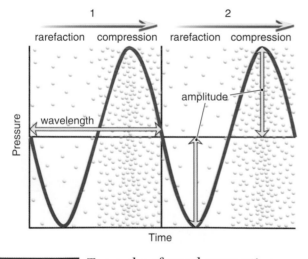

1   2
rarefaction   compression   rarefaction   compression

amplitude

wavelength

Pressure

Time

| Figure 2.1 | Two cycles of sound propagating through a medium. |

Figure 2.2 Some sound is reflected (echoed) when the ultrasound pulse encounters an interface between tissues with different values of acoustic impedence. The remaining unreflected sound energy continues on (through-transmission).

Figure 2.3 Reflection and through-transmission at sequential acoustic interfaces. The greater the difference in acoustic impedence, the greater the amplitude of the reflection.

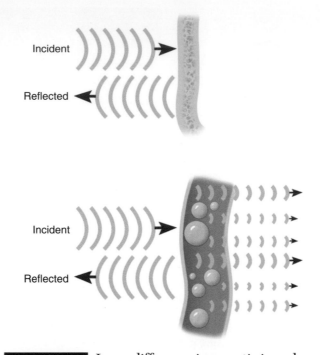

| Figure 2.4 | Large difference in acoustic impedence at an interface results in a bright reflection and much reduced through-transmission, making it difficult (or impossible) to image tissues beyond the interface. |

Attenuation

As US pulses propagate through tissues there is progressive loss of energy, referred to as attenuation. **Attenuation** is mainly due to tissue absorption of sound energy (converted to heat) plus additional energy loss due to reflection and scattering. The absolute amount of attenuation varies in different tissues and is directly proportional to frequency: as frequency increases, attenuation increases. This means that higher-frequency US pulses are limited to imaging relatively superficial structures, whereas lower frequencies must be used to image deeper structures (e.g., general abdominal imaging).

Fluids

Fluids such as blood, bile, and urine produce a very small amount of attenuation compared with other tissues. For this reason, a full urinary bladder provides a useful insonation window for suprapubic transabdominal imaging of pelvic structures, such as the uterus, ovaries, and rectouterine pouch in females or the seminal vesicles and prostate gland in males.

ACOUSTIC SHADOWING AND INCREASED THROUGH-TRANSMISSION FIG. 2.5

Because sound energy propagates through fluid with minimal attenuation compared with soft tissues, more sound energy is transmitted to the tissues deep to a fluid collection (compared with the nonfluid sound path on either side of the fluid collection). As a result, there is noticeably increased **echogenicity** in the tissues deep to fluid collections, referred to as increased through-transmission. The presence of increased through-transmission helps to confirm that an anechoic space is indeed fluid filled.

Acoustic Shadowing
Behind high-attenuation structures like bone or calcified stones

Dirty Shadowing
Behind gas/air

Increased Through-transmission
Behind a fluid-filled structure

Fluid path through large vessel (IVC) and increased through-transmission

Bowel gas reflection and dirty shadowing

Vertebral body reflection and acoustic shadowing

 Figure 2.5 Clean acoustic shadowing (bone or calcified structures), dirty acoustic shadowing (gas collections), and increased through-transmission (fluid-filled spaces). IVC, inferior vena cava.

Bone

Bone presents a substantial barrier to US transmission because of attenuation due to reflection and absorption of sound energy by compact bone. As a result, there is a bright echo from bone surfaces with a clean-edged dark acoustic shadow in the US image field beyond (see Figure 2.5).

Air

Air presents a virtually impenetrable barrier to US imaging because of reflection, reverberation, and scattering. Normally aerated lungs cannot be imaged with US, which can produce images only to the depth of pleura unless pathological fluid has filled the alveolar spaces. Gas in the gastrointestinal (GI) tract presents a major barrier in abdominal ultrasonography. In elective abdominal US imaging, patients are instructed to fast for 6 to 12 hours before their appointments to minimize GI gas. For non-elective abdominal US, a variety of tricks and techniques must be learned to obtain useful images when there is bowel gas present obscuring the region of interest. Gas (GI gas or pathological gas collections, such as tissue emphysema, pneumobilia, and necrotizing fasciitis) produces a bright reflection and hazy gray-to-black shadowing with indistinct edges (*dirty* shadowing) beyond the reflection (see Figure 2.5).

Ultrasound Probes

Piezoelectric Effect

PIEZOELECTRIC EFFECT FIG. 2.6

The piezoelectric effect is the conversion (**transduction**) of a mechanical force (such as sound) to electricity by deforming a piezoelectric crystal. Deformation of piezoelectric crystals results in a net charge across the crystal. As sound wave pressures compress and expand the crystal, the charge magnitude and polarity alternates.

"REVERSE" PIEZOELECTRIC EFFECT AND US PULSE PRODUCTION FIG. 2.7

The piezoelectric effect also works in reverse, converting electrical energy into sound energy, through alternating compression/rarefaction (i.e., vibration) when an alternating voltage is applied across a piezoelectric crystal.

Probe Transducers and Crystal Arrays

US transducers are made up of multiple piezoelectric crystals arranged in groups called arrays, housed within the US probe. US **probe transducers** both convert electricity into sound, producing the pulse that is directed into tissues, and convert sound (echoes reflected back to the probe from the tissues) into electrical signals that are then filtered and amplified to form an anatomical image of the slice being examined.

Because of the direct relationship between frequency and attenuation, higher-frequency probes (which produce better image detail) cannot be used for US applications that require deeper penetration into tissues, such as cardiac and general abdominal imaging. Thus, different US applications require probes with different fundamental frequencies and different configurations of crystal arrays.

US PROBE CRYSTAL ARRAYS: INTERACTING SOUND WAVELETS FIG. 2.8

Essentially all contemporary US probes for medical imaging contain arrays of lead-zirconate-titanate (PZT) crystals, which are electronically activated sequentially to steer and focus the US beam. This is a complex topic, but, briefly, each individual crystal in an array produces a point source wave (Huygen wavelet) when excited by an electrical pulse.

STEERING AND FOCUSING US "BEAMS" FIG. 2.9

The wavelets interact with each other constructively and destructively—peaks add up with peaks, troughs subtract from peaks, and troughs subtract from troughs—to produce a wave front with a size, shape, and direction. When crystals in an array are excited simultaneously, the wavelet interference patterns result in a wave front parallel to the array/probe face. When the array elements are excited with a sequential delay from one side to the other, the wavelets and their resulting interference patterns result in a wave-front steering. When the array elements are excited with a peripheral to central delay, the wavelet interference patterns result in a wave-front focusing: the resulting pulse is the narrowest at some depth (focal depth) and wider before and beyond the focal depth.

PULSE/ECHO SCAN LINES FIG. 2.10

Each pulse transmitted by the transducer crystal array (many thousands of pulses are

Compressing force

Expanding force

Piezoelectric crystal

+ + + + +

- - - - -

- - - - -

+ + + + +

Figure 2.6 Mechanical deformation of piezoelectric crystals results in a net charge across the crystal.

transmitted each second to form the display image) is both steered and focused. The display image is formed one scan line at a time, and a pulse is transmitted along one of a thousand or so sequential scan lines from one side of the image to the other. The next pulse along the next scan line is not transmitted until all of the echoes from the previous pulse have had time to return to the transducer. The listening time is calculated from the depth setting using average soft tissue sound velocity (0.154 cm/μs). When echoes from the last scan line on the far side of the image have returned to the transducer, the process begins again. This must be repeated 30 to 40 times every second (screen refresh rate or frame rate) for real-time motion to appear undelayed and natural in the screen image. The transducer is in pulse mode less than 1% of the time and in listening mode more than 99% of the time in a typical scan. Some probe arrays produce sector (pie-shaped) images, whereas others produce linear/rectangular images. Sector images become progressively wider with depth, whereas linear images are the same width from the surface to the deepest part of the image.

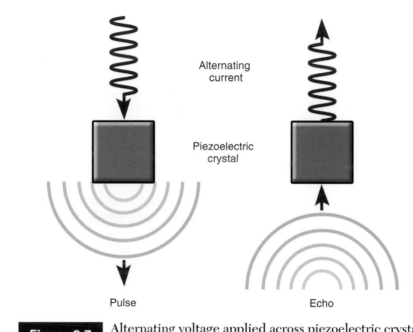

Alternating current

Piezoelectric crystal

Pulse

Echo

Figure 2.7 Alternating voltage applied across piezoelectric crystals produces the ultrasound pulse. Echoes returning to the probe mechanically deform the crystals producing electrical current, which is analyzed for image forming.

Figure 2.8 Point-source sound waves (Huygen wavelets) interacting.

Near field

Focal depth

Far field

Figure 2.9 Phased excitation of array crystals steers and focuses the ultrasound beam.

Linear

Sector

Figure 2.10 Images are formed 1 scan line at a time, proceeding sequentially from one side of the probe face to the other, repeated many times per second.

Producing an Image

The speed of sound in soft tissue is assumed to be a constant 1540 m/s (0.154 cm/μs). If, for example, the scan depth is set to 5 cm, the time required for each scan line is 65 μs. The total path length is 10 cm (5 cm from probe to depth setting and 5 cm back for returning echoes), so time = 10 cm/0.154 cm/μs = 65 μs. If there is a tissue reflector in the image at a depth of 2 cm, the total path length would be 4 cm (2 cm from the probe to the reflector and 2 cm back to the probe) and the echo from that reflector would return to the transducer at 26 μs (4 cm/0.154 cm/μs = 26 μs). Stated from the point of view of the US unit, any echo from a scan line reaching the transducer at 26 μs is displayed in the image at a depth of 2 cm.

**FORMING IMAGES:
SCAN LINES
ECHO RETURN TIME
AND AMPLITUDE
FIG. 2.11**

Putting it together, each tissue reflector in the image is displayed (1) in side-to-side position based on the line being scanned when the echo reaches the transducer, (2) at some depth determined by the time

when the echo returns, and (3) at some gray-scale value from black to white based on the intensity (**amplitude**) of the echo.

**BEAM WIDTH:
DISPLAY OF SMALL
REFLECTORS
AND SPATIAL
RESOLUTION
FIG. 2.12**

Lastly, **spatial resolution** is the ability to distinguish and display small objects that are close together as separate in space. Small objects are displayed as the width of the beam at the depth they are located (lateral smearing artifact). Lateral (side-to-side) resolution, for example, is the ability to distinguish and display 2 small reflectors that are close together perpendicular to the direction of the US pulse as separate objects. Lateral resolution varies with beam width, increasing as beam width decreases. Beam width is largely determined by the frequency and focal depth. Higher-frequency probes produce narrower beams and, therefore, have better lateral resolution. Lateral resolution is always best at the focal depth, where the beam is the narrowest.

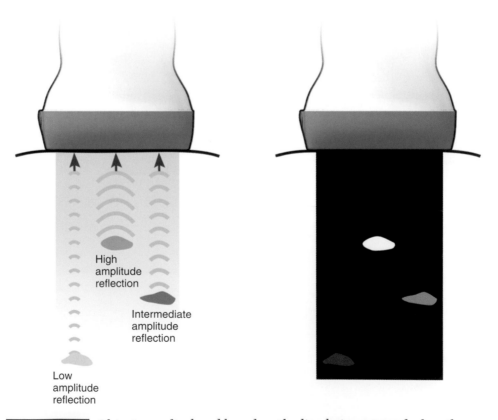

High
amplitude
reflection

Intermediate
amplitude
reflection

Low
amplitude
reflection

Figure 2.11 Objects are displayed based on the line being scanned when the echo returns, the time when the echo returns, and the amplitude of the echo.

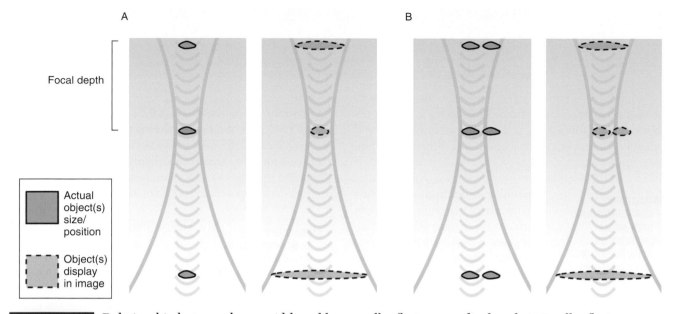

Figure 2.12 Relationship between beam width and how small reflectors are displayed. A, Small reflectors are displayed as the width of the beam at the depth they are located (lateral smearing artifact). B, Lateral resolution (the ability to distinguish side-by-side small reflectors) is best near the focal depth, where the beam is the narrowest.

Specular Reflection and Diffuse Reflection

In considering how various tissues/structures appear in US images, it is useful to think of 2 broad categories of sound wave reflection, specular reflection and diffuse reflection (scattering).

ANISOTROPY: CHANGING SOUND PATH ANGLE CHANGES US APPEARANCE OF SOME OBJECTS FIG. 2.13

Specular reflection occurs when sound waves encounter a smooth surface or a smooth interface between 2 tissues with different acoustic properties. This type of reflection is responsible for the hyperechoic edges/interfaces seen in US images and for the bright appearance of fibrous structures, such as tendons, ligaments, and organ capsules. Specular reflection is best for image forming when the surface or interface is perpendicular to the path of the sound pulses. When sound pulses encounter a specular reflector, its appearance changes as its angle changes relative to the sound path. When the path is perpendicular to a specular reflector, most of the echoed energy returns to the probe to be detected for image forming, so the reflector appears as a bright white (hyperechoic) line in the US display. When sound pulses encounter the same reflector at an angle sufficiently different from 90 degrees, the sound energy is reflected such that none (or only a small proportion) of the echoes return to the probe transducer to form an image—the same reflector appears dark (hypoechoic/anechoic) in the US display.

ANISOTROPY DEMONSTRATED IN A CURVING TENDON FIG. 2.14

This artifact, in which the same reflector appears as bright when the angle of insonation is close to perpendicular and appears as dark when imaged from a different angle, is referred to as anisotropy. In the US image shown in Figure 2.14, fascicles of collagen in the tendon of the infraspinatus muscle act as specular reflectors, giving the characteristic fibrillar appearance of multiple thin bright lines for the region of the tendon that is roughly perpendicular to the probe face. As the tendon curves over the humeral head (and away from perpendicular to the US beam), the bright fibrillar lines darken and disappear owing to anisotropy.

 Anisotropy—the same reflector can appear as hyperechoic or hypoechoic/anechoic, depending on the angle of the ultrasound beam.

SCATTERING AND "SPECKLED" APPEARANCE OF MANY TISSUES FIG. 2.15

When sound waves encounter elements within tissues that are irregular or "bumpy" to sound waves (irregularities that are smaller than the wavelength of the US), **diffuse reflection** or scattering occurs. The scattered sound waves interfere with one another in complex patterns, giving rise to the speckled echo-texture of tissues such as liver, spleen, kidney, and myocardium. Because the scattered reflections (and resulting interference patterns) occur in multiple directions, the US appearance of these tissues is relatively unchanging, regardless of the angle of insonation.

Hyperechoic fibrillar appearance disappears due to anisotropy

Figure 2.14 Ultrasound image of a tendon demonstrating anisotropy artifact.

Figure 2.15 Diffuse reflection (scattering) results in interference patterns that produce the speckled echo appearance of many organs. The appearance of these tissues is largely unaffected by the angle of the ultrasound beam.

Bioeffects of Ultrasound Energy

Because tissue absorption of sound energy is the most important source of attenuation, it also has implications for the health/safety of US imaging. Absorbed sound energy is converted to heat, so there are potential thermal **bioeffects** on tissues. The potential for bioeffects vary with the duration of exposure to sound energy (total scanning time); specific amount of tissue attenuation (more attenuation = more thermal effect, so tissues such as bone are more susceptible); location in the scan field (tissues that are superficial and nearer the focal zone have the highest exposure); frequency (higher frequencies = more attenuation = greater thermal effect); pulse transmission power; and pulse duration/pulse repetition frequency (some scan modes, such as Doppler mode, require higher pulse repetition frequencies and therefore result in higher exposure).

3

Back

Lumbar Spine

Review of the Anatomy

Lumbar Vertebrae

The 5 lumbar **vertebrae**, similar to all typical vertebrae, consist of a body anteriorly and a vertebral arch posteriorly. The vertebral arch consists of right and left pedicles that attach the arch to the vertebral body and right and left laminae that fuse in the midline and form the bony roof of the vertebral canal. The transverse processes project laterally from the junction of the pedicles and laminae, and immediately posterior to this point, articular processes project superiorly and inferiorly. The articular surfaces of the superior articular processes face posteromedially, and those of the inferior articular processes face anterolaterally. Zygapophyseal (facet) joints are formed between the inferior articular process of the vertebra above and the superior articular process of the vertebra below. Because of the orientation of lumbar articular processes, the joint space itself is oriented obliquely about halfway between the frontal and sagittal planes. The spinous process projects posteriorly (and slightly inferiorly) in the midline from the junction of the right and left laminae. The posterior surface of the vertebral body, the pedicles, and the laminae form the borders of a bony vertebral foramen in each vertebra.

Adjacent vertebral bodies are joined by intervertebral discs as well as anterior and posterior longitudinal ligaments. Ligamenta flava join the laminae of adjacent vertebrae. The interspinous and supraspinous ligaments join the spinous processes. Zygapophyseal joints between the inferior and superior articular processes are the only synovial joints between adjacent vertebrae.

Spinal Canal

The spinal cord, including the conus medullaris and cauda equina, plus the surrounding spinal meninges are housed within the vertebral **(spinal) canal**, which is formed by the aligned vertebral foramina and associated soft tissues, including the ligamenta flava, intervertebral discs, and the posterior longitudinal ligament. The spinal dura mater is separated from the interior of the canal by a variable amount of extradural fat and venous plexus. The meningeal and neural contents of the lumbar spinal canal include the dural sac, conus medullaris, cauda equina, filum terminale, and lumbar cistern of subarachnoid space.

Throughout most of the vertebral column, the laminae and spinous processes of adjacent vertebrae overlap to the extent that there is a more or less continuous bony covering of the spinal canal posteriorly. In the lumbar region, however, relatively large spaces between adjacent vertebral arches appear, such that there are gaps (**interlaminar spaces**) in the bony covering of the spinal canal, which are filled by the ligamenta flava. The size of these gaps increases with flexion, and they provide soft tissue windows for ultrasound imaging of the lumbar spinal canal and its contents.

Deep Back Muscles

The deep fascia of the back and back muscles related to the lumbar vertebrae include the thoracolumbar fascia (fused to the aponeurotic tendon of origin of latissimus dorsi), erector spinae, multifidus, and psoas major muscles. The erector spinae muscle is covered by the thoracolumbar fascia (posterior layer), and most of its muscle mass in the lumbar region is seen overlying (posterior to) the transverse processes of lumbar vertebrae. The multifidus muscle is well developed in the lumbar region and occupies the space adjacent to the spinous processes and posterior surfaces of the laminae and articular processes/zygapophyseal joints of lumbar vertebrae. The psoas major muscle is a muscle of the posterior abdominal wall that occupies the space adjacent to the bodies and anterior surfaces of transverse processes of lumbar vertebrae.

Technique

For all of the views described in detail as follows, the patient should be positioned either (1) sitting sideways on the examination table leaning forward (flexing the lumbar region as much as possible to increase the size of the interlaminar spaces) with the forearms resting on the thighs or (2) lying prone on the examination table with a pillow/bolster placed under the lower part of the abdomen (positioned to flex the lumbar region as much as possible). Care should be taken to ensure that the spinous processes are aligned in the sagittal plane with as little tilt/rotation to one side or the other as possible. In clinical settings (e.g., for lumbar puncture or epidural anesthesia) the lateral decubitus position with the patient curled into a "fetal position" is also commonly used, but this position tends to be difficult for inexperienced examiners. For orientation purposes, palpate and mark the spinous process of L4 in the midline at the intercristal line (a line interconnecting the highest points on the iliac crests).

**INTERLAMINAR SPACE
THECAL SAC**
Transverse
FIG. 3.2

Using a low frequency (2-5 MHz) curved array probe, place the probe face transversely over the L4 spinous process. Identify the reflection and acoustic shadow of the spinous process, and position it in the center of the image. Carefully adjust the probe position until the spinous process and laminae can be seen. Look for the thin anechoic/hypoechoic lines representing the zygapophyseal joint spaces at the lateral extent of the laminae on both

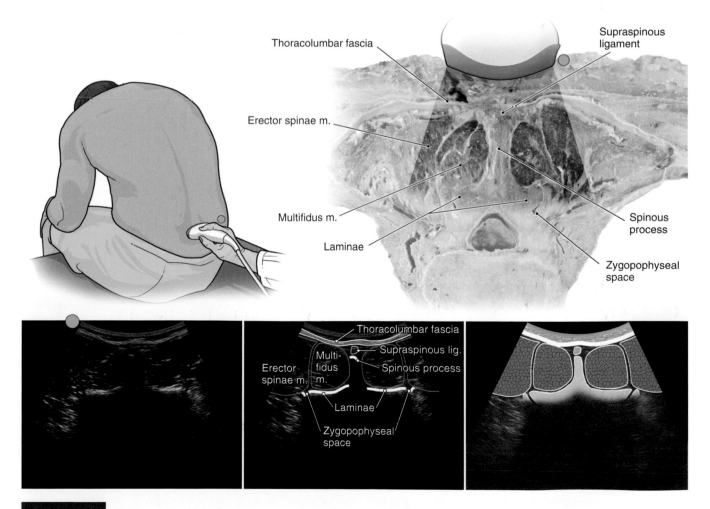

Figure 3.1 Transverse view of spinous process and laminae with overlying deep back muscles.

sides. Identify the skin and superficial fascia, the hyperechoic thoracolumbar fascia, and the "starry sky" appearance of the multifidus and erector spinae muscles.

TRANSVERSE PROCESSES
Longitudinal
FIG. 3.3

Carefully slide the probe slightly inferiorly until the reflection/acoustic shadow of the spinous process disappears, replaced with the hypoechoic interspinous ligament. The laminae also fall away as the articular processes come into view, 1 to 2 cm deeper in the image. The interlaminar space can be identified as the gap between the medial edges of the articular processes. Two hyperechoic bands, the posterior and anterior complexes, should then be identified. The posterior complex, which spans the interlaminar space immediately superficial to the articular processes, represents the combined reflections of the ligamentum flavum, the extradural space, and the posterior

aspect of the dura mater. The anterior complex, the hyperechoic band that is seen 1 to 2 cm deep to the posterior complex, represents the combined reflections of the anterior aspect of the dura mater, the extradural space, and the posterior longitudinal ligament. The anterior complex is visible only when the probe is over the interlaminar space (otherwise hidden in acoustic shadow of the bony vertebral arch structures). Between the posterior and anterior complexes, the contents of the thecal sac (lumbar cistern and cauda equina) can be visualized as an oval-shaped anechoic/hypoechoic space.

ARTICULAR PROCESSES
Longitudinal
FIG. 3.4

Remaining at the L4/L5 level, place the probe along the long axis of the spine a short distance (3-4 cm) lateral to the midline, with the probe marker facing superiorly. Adjust the probe position until 2 or 3 transverse

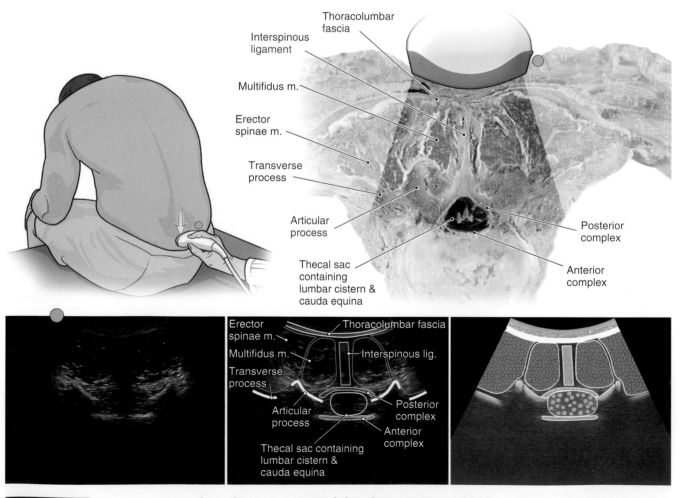

Figure 3.2 Transverse view of interlaminar space and thecal sac containing lumbar cistern and cauda equina. Posterior complex: ligamentum flavum, extradural fat, and posterior aspect of dura mater. Anterior complex: anterior aspect of dura mater, extradural fat, and posterior longitudinal ligament.

processes can be identified as the short curved hyperechoic lines deep to erector spinae muscle, with their characteristic "finger-like" acoustic shadows. Between the acoustic shadows of successive transverse processes, the psoas major muscle can be seen with its prominent hyperechoic striations. The parietal peritoneum can be identified as the hyperechoic line at the deep surface of psoas major. Respiratory movement of intraperitoneal structures deep to this line can usually be seen.

LAMINAE INTERLAMINAR SPACES
Longitudinal
FIG. 3.5

Next, slide the probe a short distance medially until a continuous line of short bony humps appears, deep to muscle. These are the overlapping articular processes of successive vertebrae, commonly referred to as the "articular column" in ultrasound (US) imaging. The multifidus is the main muscle mass overlying the articular column in the lumbar region.

After identifying the articular column, tilt the probe face slightly medially (so that the US beam is traveling from lateral to medial, from the skin surface to deeper structures) until the laminae and interlaminar spaces of successive vertebrae come into view. The laminae are seen as hyperechoic lines that are tilted relative to the skin surface such that their superior edges are deeper than their inferior edges, giving an overall sawtooth appearance. Between successive laminae and their acoustic shadows, the posterior complex, contents of the thecal sac, and the anterior complex can be seen.

Thoracolumbar fascia

Erector spinae m.

Transverse processes

Intertransverse muscles & ligaments

Psoas m.

Parietal peritoneum

Thoracolumbar fascia

Transverse processes

Erector spinae m.

Intertransverse muscles & ligs.

Psoas m.

Psoas m.

Parietal peritoneum

Figure 3.3 Longitudinal (parasagittal) view of erector spinae muscle, transverse processes, and psoas major muscle.

CLINICAL APPLICATIONS

These techniques can be used for evaluating and accurately measuring the anatomy of the lumbar spine and associated ligaments, extradural space, and lumbar cistern before diagnostic lumbar puncture or administration of spinal or epidural anesthesia. For example, the depth from the skin surface to the ligamentum flavum, epidural space, dura mater, and intrathecal space can be accurately measured using the caliper function of the US equipment and vertebral levels can be ascertained and marked on the skin surface in patients with confusing or difficult anatomy. These techniques can also be used for US-guided needle advancement and insertion during lumbar puncture and/or administration of spinal/epidural anesthesia or zygapophyseal joint injection.

Thoracolumbar fascia

Multifidus m.

Overlapping articular processes of successive vertebrae (articular column)

Thoracolumbar fascia

Multifidus m.

Overlapping articular processes of successive vertebrae (articular column)

Figure 3.4 Longitudinal (parasagittal) view of articular processes with overlying multifidus muscle.

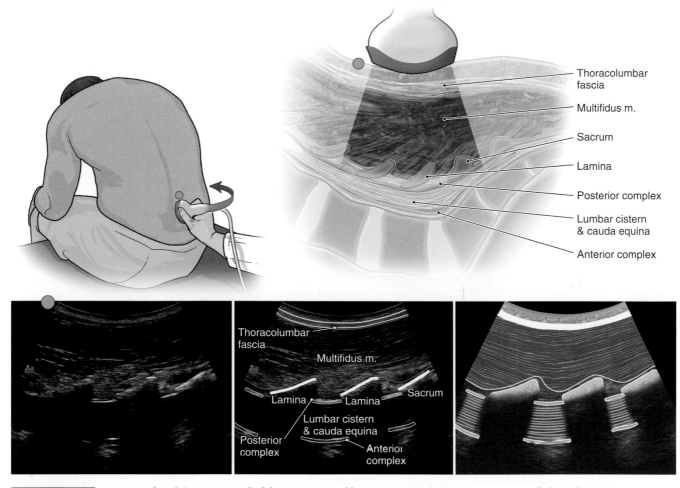

Thoracolumbar fascia

Multifidus m.

Sacrum

Lamina

Posterior complex

Lumbar cistern & cauda equina

Anterior complex

Figure 3.5 Longitudinal (parasagittal oblique) view of laminae, interlaminar spaces, and thecal sac with overlying multifidus muscle. Posterior complex: ligamentum flavum, extradural fat, and posterior aspect of dura mater. Anterior complex: anterior aspect of dura mater, extradural fat, and posterior longitudinal ligament.

4

Upper Limb

Brachial Plexus

Review of the Anatomy

The brachial plexus is the source of innervation for the upper limb. The plexus forms in the neck from the primary ventral rami of spinal nerves C5 through T1, referred to as the roots of the plexus. The roots emerge from their respective intervertebral foramina into the scalene interval, a narrow space between anterior and middle scalene muscles. Typically, C5 and C6 roots combine to form the upper trunk, C7 root continues as the middle trunk, and the C8 and T1 roots combine to form the lower trunk. The trunks continue toward the root of the neck, where each divides into an anterior and a posterior division. The divisions then cross the first rib just lateral to the subclavian artery, between the anterior and middle scalene tendons (which insert on the first rib). The anterior and posterior divisions recombine to form the cords of the plexus as they pass through the space between the first rib, clavicle, and superior margin of the scapula (axillary inlet or cervicoaxillary canal) into the axilla. As it passes beyond the lateral margin of the first rib, the subclavian artery becomes the axillary artery. The axillary vein is medial/inferior to the artery and crosses the first rib on the medial side of the anterior scalene tendon (i.e., not through the scalene interval). In their course through the axilla, the divisions, cords and branches of the plexus, and the axillary vessels are deep to the pectoralis muscles. The axillary artery is described as having 3 parts: the first part is superior/medial to the pectoralis minor muscle, the second part is posterior/deep to the pectoralis minor muscle, and the third part is inferior/lateral to pectoralis minor. As the cords form from the divisions, they come to surround the second part of the artery and are named for their relationship to the artery in this position: the lateral cord is lateral/superior to the artery, the medial cord is medial/inferior to the artery (between the artery and vein), and the posterior cord is posterior/deep to the artery.

Pectoralis Muscles

Pectoralis major is a large fan-shaped muscle that originates along the medial third of the clavicle, the surface of the sternum, and the first 7 costal cartilages. It inserts through a ribbonlike tendon onto the lateral lip of the intertubercular groove. The pectoralis minor muscle, deep to pectoralis major, is a small triangular muscle originating from the surfaces of ribs 3 to 5 and inserting on the medial aspect of the coracoid process of the scapula.

Technique

Roots, Trunks, and Divisions

SCALENE INTERVAL ROOTS AND TRUNKS
Transverse
FIG. 4.1

The patient should be supine on the examination table with the head rotated slightly to the contralateral side. Position the probe transversely a few centimeters above the medial third of the clavicle, over the lower part of the sternocleidomastoid muscle. Adjust the probe position as needed to identify the following structures deep to sternocleidomastoid (for additional information see Chapter 9 Neck and Face), from medial to lateral: the common carotid artery, the internal jugular vein, and the anterior scalene muscle. Slide the probe laterally until the internal jugular vein is just visible at the medial aspect of the image. In this position, identify the anterior and middle scalene muscles and the thin space between them, the scalene interval. Slide the probe superiorly and inferiorly over the scalene interval while adjusting the probe tilt/angle until 2 or 3 large bundles of nerve tissue can be identified in the interval (in many patients, because of the oblique course of the roots/trunks relative to the surface of the neck and resulting anisotropy/artifact, the roots/trunks can only be seen as discrete hypoechoic ovals, sometimes referred to as the "traffic-light" sign). The C5, C6, and C7 roots are the most anterior nerve bundles in the interval, and the lower parts of the plexus (C8 and T1 roots) are difficult to definitively image in this location.

ROOT OF THE NECK TRUNKS AND DIVISIONS
Transverse
FIG. 4.2

From the interscalene view of the brachial plexus, simultaneously slide the probe inferiorly toward the supraclavicular fossa while tilting the probe face inferiorly until the view is nearly coronal. While repositioning/tilting the probe, keep the bundles of

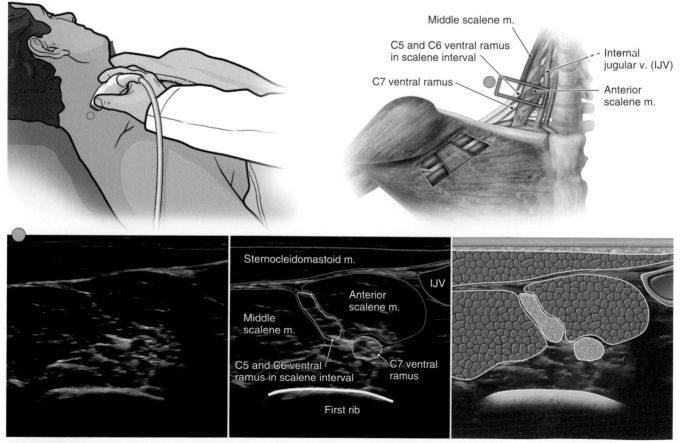

Middle scalene m.

C5 and C6 ventral ramus in scalene interval

C7 ventral ramus

Internal jugular v. (IJV)

Anterior scalene m.

Sternocleidomastoid m.

IJV

Anterior scalene m.

Middle scalene m.

C5 and C6 ventral ramus in scalene interval

C7 ventral ramus

First rib

Figure 4.1 Transverse view of the roots and trunks of the brachial plexus in the scalene interval. IJV, internal jugular vein.

nerve tissue of the plexus near the center of the image and look for the appearance of the pulsating subclavian artery and the hyperechoic reflection (and acoustic shadow) of the first rib. The trunks/divisions of the plexus appear as a very large stack of nerve tissue bundles draped over the first rib in contact with the lateral surface of the subclavian artery. The lower trunk (combined C8 and T1 roots) is inferiorly positioned, in contact with the first rib between the middle scalene muscle/tendon and the subclavian artery.

Cords

AXILLA
CORDS
Transverse
FIG. 4.3

The patient should be supine on the examination table with the arm resting along the side. In some patients, it may be helpful to ask them to place their hand palm up behind their head, which moves the scapula anteriorly and brings the axillary vessels into a more superficial position. By palpation, locate the positions of the coracoid process and the xiphisternal junction. Place the probe along the diagonal line connecting these landmarks, just below the tip of the coracoid process (probe orientation marker toward the coracoid). Identify the pectoralis major muscle in oblique/transverse view and the pectoralis minor muscle viewed in its longitudinal axis. Deep to the pectoralis minor, identify the pulsating axillary artery (second part) and adjust the probe position, pressure, and tilt as necessary to identify the axillary vein immediately medial/inferior to the artery and to obtain a true transverse view (circular rather than oval profile) of the artery. Three hyperechoic nerve bundles should be visible near the artery. The lateral cord is seen just lateral/superior to the artery. The posterior cord is immediately deep to the artery. The medial cord is medial/inferior to the artery, situated between the artery and the vein.

CLINICAL APPLICATIONS

These techniques are most commonly used to guide needles (or catheters) safely into position for infiltration of local anesthetic agents around the components of the brachial plexus to establish regional anesthesia during upper limb surgery and/or for pain control in the postoperative period.

Plexus blocks in the scalene interval are referred to as interscalene blocks. Blocks in the root of the neck are referred to as supraclavicular blocks. Blocks of the cords in the axilla are called infraclavicular blocks.

Each of these sites carries its own set of advantages, disadvantages, and indications for use.

- Interscalene blocks reliably anesthetize the upper arm and shoulder but often miss the C8 and T1 roots, thereby failing to anesthetize the ulnar side of the arm, forearm, and hand.

- Because the nerve trunks/divisions are packed closely together in the root of the neck, supraclavicular blocks reliably produce virtually complete upper limb anesthesia. However, because of the proximity of the lung apex and subclavian artery to the trunks of the plexus in this location, there is risk of puncturing the lung and producing a pneumothorax or arterial puncture and intravascular injection of local anesthetic.

Infraclavicular blocks (plexus cords) produce reliable anesthesia of the distal two-thirds of the arm, forearm, wrist, and hand. These blocks are often used for surgeries of the upper limb distal to and including the elbow. In addition, there is little risk for puncturing the lung and producing a pneumothorax as compared with supraclavicular blocks.

Middle scalene m.

Anterior scalene m.

Trunks of plexus

Subclavian a.

Omohyoid m. inferior belly

Sternocleidomastoid m.

Subclavian a.

Trunks of plexus

Middle scalene m.

Anterior scalene m.

First rib

Cupula

Figure 4.2 Transverse view of the trunks and divisions of the brachial plexus alongside the subclavian artery in the root of the neck.

Axillary v.
Medial cord
Axillary a.
Lateral cord

Pectoralis minor m.
Pectoralis major m.

Pectoralis major m.

Pectoralis minor m.

Lateral cord

Axillary a.

Axillary v.

Posterior cord

Medial cord

Figure 4.3 Transverse view of the cords of the brachial plexus surrounding the axillary artery, deep to the pectoralis major and minor muscles.

Shoulder

Review of the Anatomy

Bones

The bones of the shoulder are the scapula, the proximal humerus, and the clavicle.

Scapula

The scapula is a large, flat, triangular bone. The scapular spine projects from its posterior surface, dividing the posterior scapula into a supraspinous and an infraspinous fossa. The spine expands at its lateral end into the acromion process, which forms much of the bony roof over the glenohumeral joint, the synovial ball and socket joint between the head of the humerus and the relatively small, shallow, glenoid cavity at the lateral angle of the scapula. The depth and circumference of the glenoid cavity are increased by a fibrocartilaginous collar, the glenoid labrum. The fingerlike coracoid process that projects anteriorly and laterally from the superior margin of the scapula, together with the acromion and the intervening coracoacromial ligament, makes up the coracoacromial arch, which roofs over the humeral head and glenohumeral joint. The space between the deep surface of the arch and the humeral head is the subacromial space.

Proximal Humerus and Glenohumeral Joint

From the proximal humerus, the hemispherical humeral head projects posteromedially and slightly superiorly toward the glenoid fossa of the scapula. The head is demarcated from the remainder of the proximal humerus by a narrow constriction, the anatomical neck. The greater and lesser tubercles, which serve as attachment sites for the tendons of the rotator cuff muscles, are situated at the anterior aspect of the proximal humerus, separated by the intertubercular groove.

The greater tubercle has a rounded surface that projects anterolaterally, with 3 facets (superior, middle, and inferior) for attachment of the tendons of supraspinatus, infraspinatus, and teres minor (the rotator cuff muscles originating from the posterior scapula). The lesser tubercle, projecting anteriorly and somewhat medially, has a flattened to slightly concave surface for attachment of the tendon of subscapularis (the rotator cuff muscle originating from the anterior [costal or thoracic] surface of the scapula).

The tendon of the long head of biceps brachii occupies the intertubercular groove and is stabilized in that position by the transverse humeral ligament. Superiorly, the tendon curves over the humeral head and passes through a small interval (rotator cuff interval) between the tendons of supraspinatus and subscapularis to enter the glenohumeral joint space. The rotator cuff tendons course superficially over the fibrous capsule of the glenohumeral joint to reach their insertion sites on the greater and lesser tubercles. The fibrous capsule is attached along the anatomical neck of the humerus and along the margin of the glenoid fossa, just outside the glenoid labrum.

Clavicle and Acromioclavicular Joint

The clavicle is subcutaneous throughout its length. Its medial end is attached to the sternum at the sternoclavicular joint, and its lateral end is attached to the acromion of the scapula at the acromioclavicular (AC) joint. The AC joint is a small synovial joint between the anteromedial surface of the acromion and the lateral end of the clavicle. The joint is enclosed by a capsule, which is reinforced by a thickening along its subcutaneous superior surface, the AC ligament.

Muscles

Deltoid

The deltoid muscle, which forms the normal rounded contour of the shoulder, is immediately superficial to the rotator cuff tendons and the tendon of the long head of biceps brachii. The deltoid muscle has a wide U-shaped origin from the scapular spine, acromion, and lateral third of the clavicle and tapers to its insertion on the deltoid tubercle at the lateral lip of the intertubercular groove near the mid-diaphysis of the humerus.

Supraspinatus

The supraspinatus muscle originates from the supraspinous fossa, and its tendon passes through the subacromial space to insert on the superior facet of the greater tubercle. The subacromial bursa separates the tendon from the deep surface of the acromion and coracoacromial arch. Beyond the subacromial space, the tendon is separated from the deep surface of the deltoid muscle by a continuation of the subdeltoid bursa (continuous with the subacromial bursa) and a thin plane of subdeltoid/peribursal fat.

Infraspinatus and Teres Minor

The infraspinatus and teres minor muscles originate from the infraspinous fossa. Their tendons pass beneath the posterior edge of the acromion and over the posterior aspect of the glenohumeral joint and humeral head to insert on the middle and inferior facets of the greater tubercle.

These muscles and their tendons are separated from the overlying deltoid muscle by a thin layer of subdeltoid fat and fascia.

Subscapularis

The subscapularis muscle originates from the anterior surface of the scapula, and its tendon passes through the subcoracoid space inferior to the coracoid process and deep to the coracobrachialis and short head of biceps brachii muscles, then over the anteromedial aspect of the glenohumeral joint and humeral head to insert on the lesser tubercle. Beyond the subcoracoid space the tendon is immediately deep to the deltoid muscle and subdeltoid fat and fascia.

Technique

Tendon of the Long Head of Biceps Brachii

INTERTUBERCULAR GROOVE
BICEPS BRACHII
LONG HEAD TENDON
Transverse
FIG. 4.4

The patient should be seated with the elbow flexed to 90 degrees and the supinated forearm resting on the thigh. Standing behind the patient, position the probe (linear high frequency) transverse to the anterior surface of the proximal humerus with the probe marker pointed laterally. Deep to the deltoid muscle, identify the greater and lesser tubercles and the intervening intertubercular groove. The tendon of the long head of biceps brachii should appear as a hyperechoic oval within the groove. Although a tendon sheath extends along the tendon a short distance from the glenohumeral joint, it is not normally seen unless there are inflammatory changes such as tenosynovitis or joint effusion. Tilting/fanning the probe alters the appearance of the tendon from hyperechoic to hypoechoic/anechoic (because of anisotropy). A thin hyperechoic band of dense connective tissue, the transverse humeral ligament, should be seen spanning the groove just anterior to the tendon and blending with connective tissue along the surfaces of the tubercles.

INTERTUBERCULAR GROOVE
BICEPS BRACHII
LONG HEAD TENDON
Longitudinal
FIG. 4.5

Keeping the tendon in view in the center of the image, rotate the probe 90 degrees (probe marker facing superiorly) to obtain a longitudinal view. Owing to anisotropy, the tendon "disappears" superiorly as it curves over the humerus into the joint space.

Deltoid m.
Greater tubercle
Tendon of biceps brachii long head
Lesser tubercle
Humerus
Subscapularis tendon

Deltoid m.
Transverse humeral ligament
Greater tubercle
Intertubercular groove
Humerus
Tendon of biceps brachii long head
Lesser tubercle
Subscapularis tendon

Figure 4.4 Transverse view of the tendon of the long head of biceps brachii in the intertubercular groove of the humerus.

Subscapularis

SUBSCAPULARIS TENDON
Longitudinal
FIG. 4.6

The patient should be seated with the elbow flexed to 90 degrees and the forearm supinated as before. Placing the probe transverse to the anterior aspect of the proximal humerus, once again identify the lesser tubercle and externally rotate the patient's arm. Deep to the deltoid muscle and subdeltoid fat and fascia, the tendon of subscapularis will come into view (in the longitudinal axis of the tendon). Identify the tendon as it curves over the humeral head from the subcoracoid space to its tapered lateral end where it inserts onto the lesser tubercle.

SUBSCAPULARIS TENDON
Transverse
FIG. 4.7

Rotate the probe 90 degrees (probe marker facing superiorly) to view the tendon across its longitudinal axis. Slide the probe medially a very short distance until several hyperechoic tendon bundles interspersed with hypoechoic muscle tissue (myotendinous junctions) can be identified.

Supraspinatus Tendon

GREATER TUBERCLE SUPRASPINATUS TENDON
Longitudinal
FIG. 4.8

The patient's limb should be in the "hand in the back pocket" (modified Crass) position with the palm over the lower back and the elbow pointing posteriorly. This position extends/hyperextends and externally rotates the humerus, bringing the supraspinatus tendon out of the subacromial space. Place the probe over the anterior lateral corner of the shoulder just distal to the acromion, angled approximately midway between the sagittal and coronal planes (probe marker pointing anterolaterally) to obtain a longitudinal ("bird's beak") view of the tendon. Adjust the position of the probe until the fibrillar appearance of the tendon is clearly seen and the tapered end of the tendon at its insertion on the greater tubercle comes into view. Identify from superficial to deep: the deltoid muscle, the hyperechoic subdeltoid fat and fascia, the thin anechoic subdeltoid bursa, the supraspinatus tendon, the superior facet of the greater tubercle, the anatomical neck of the humerus, and the humeral head. Slide the probe anteriorly and posteriorly in the same orientation to view the tendon from side to side.

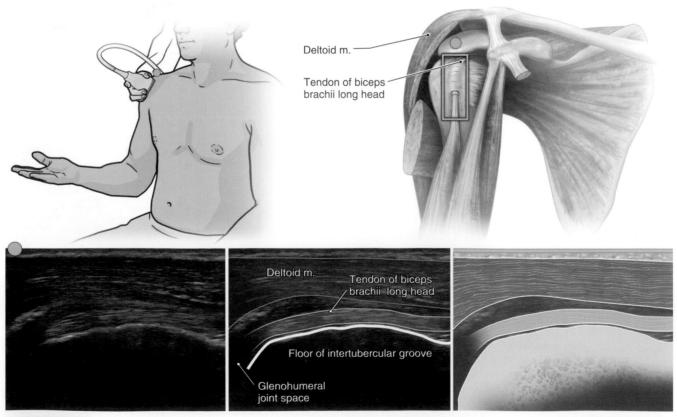

Deltoid m.

Tendon of biceps brachii long head

Deltoid m.

Tendon of biceps brachii long head

Floor of intertubercular groove

Glenohumeral joint space

| **Figure 4.5** | Longitudinal view of the tendon of the long head of biceps brachii in the intertubercular groove of the humerus. |

SUPRASPINATUS MYOTENDINOUS JUNCTION
Longitudinal
FIG. 4.9

Slide the probe along the tendon proximally (toward the patient's ear) in the same orientation until the hyperechoic surface of the acromion (and its acoustic shadow) comes into view. The myotendinous junction of supraspinatus is often visible as it emerges from the subacromial space.

ROTATOR CUFF INTERVAL SUPRASPINATUS TENDON
Transverse
FIG. 4.10

Slide the probe back distally until the tendon and its insertion are again visible. Rotate the probe 90 degrees (probe marker pointing to the right) to obtain a transverse ("tire on the rim") view of the tendon. Slide the probe medially (simultaneously adjusting the tilt/angle) until the hyperechoic oval profile of the tendon of the long head of biceps brachii in the rotator cuff interval can be identified.

Infraspinatus Tendon

INFRASPINATUS TENDON
Longitudinal
FIG. 4.11

The patient's limb should be across the chest with the fingers and palm resting on the contralateral shoulder. Place the probe on the posterior surface of the shoulder just inferior to the posterior corner of the acromion, parallel to the scapular spine. Adjust the probe position anteriorly/posteriorly in this orientation until the fibrillar appearance of the tendon is clearly seen and the tapered end at its insertion on the greater tubercle comes into view. From superficial to deep, identify the deltoid muscle, subdeltoid fat and fascia, infraspinatus tendon, greater tubercle, and head of humerus.

Tendon of biceps brachii short head
Subscapularis m. & tendon
Coracobrachialis m.
Deltoid m.
Subdeltoid fascia
Lesser tubercle
Tendon of biceps brachii long head
Greater tubercle
Head of humerus

Deltoid m.
Subdeltoid fascia
Tendon of subscapularis
Lesser tubercle
Head of humerus

Figure 4.6 Longitudinal view of the tendon of subscapularis at the lesser tubercle of the humerus.

Glenohumeral Joint and Glenoid Labrum

**GLENOHUMERAL JOINT
GLENOID LABRUM**
Transverse
FIG. 4.12

Maintaining the same patient position and probe orientation, slide the probe posteriorly (toward the midline) keeping the supraspinatus tendon in view as it becomes continuous with muscle tissue (myotendinous junction). Observe the head of the humerus as it curves toward the glenoid fossa, and look for the small bright reflection (and acoustic shadow) of the posterior rim of the glenoid process. At the glenoid rim, look for the hyperechoic triangular profile of the posterior aspect of the glenoid labrum between the articular surface of the humeral head and the infraspinatus tendon and myotendinous junction. The apex of the glenoid labrum is directed anterolaterally. Gently rotate the patient's arm externally and internally to observe the movement of the infraspinatus muscle and tendon over the posterior aspect of the glenohumeral joint and humeral head. At the posteromedial (nonmarker) edge of the image the spinoglenoid notch (inferior scapular notch) can be seen adjacent to the glenoid process.

Acromioclavicular Joint

**ACROMIOCLAVICULAR
JOINT**
Coronal
FIG. 4.13

With the patient seated and the forearm resting on the thigh, palpate along the distal clavicle to locate the small "step-off" at the AC joint. Center the probe over the joint in a coronal orientation (probe marker pointing to the right). Identify the acromion, the AC joint space, the lateral end of the clavicle, and the AC ligament.

CLINICAL APPLICATIONS

Ultrasound examination is commonly used in the evaluation of musculoskeletal injuries or degenerative disorders resulting in "painful shoulder," such as rotator cuff tendon tears or impingement (e.g., subacromial supraspinatus tendon impingement), subacromial/subdeltoid bursitis, biceps tendonitis/tenosynovitis, glenoid labrum tears and cysts, glenohumeral joint effusions, and AC joint separations. These techniques are also used to guide needles into the glenohumeral joint, AC joint, or inflamed bursae for injection of local anesthetic agents and anti-inflammatory steroids.

Deltoid m.

Tendon of subscapularis

Head of humerus/ lesser tubercle

Subdeltoid fascia   Deltoid m.

Tendon of subscapularis

Head of humerus/ lesser tubercle

Figure 4.7 Transverse view of the tendon of subscapularis with several myotendinous junctions (multipennate appearance).

Figure 4.8 Longitudinal view of the supraspinatus tendon and its insertion at the superior facet of the greater tubercle of the humerus.

Figure 4.9 Longitudinal view of the supraspinatus myotendinous junction just emerging from the subacromial space.

Deltoid m.

Tendon of supraspinatus

Head of humerus

Tendon of biceps brachii

Tendon of subscapularis

Deltoid m.

Subdeltoid fascia

Tendon of biceps brachii

Tendon of supraspinatus

Cuff interval

Head of humerus

Tendon of subscapularis

Figure 4.10 Transverse view of the supraspinatus tendon along with the tendon of the long head of biceps brachii in the rotator cuff interval.

Deltoid m.

Greater tubercle

Anatomical neck

Tendon of infraspinatus m.

Head of humerus

Articular cartilage

Deltoid m.

Subdeltoid fascia

Tendon of infraspinatus

Greater tubercle

Head of humerus

Anatomical neck

Articular cartilage

Figure 4.11 Longitudinal view of the tendon of infraspinatus and its insertion onto the middle facet of the greater tubercle of the humerus.

Deltoid m.

Glenohumeral joint capsule

Subdeltoid fascia

Infraspinatus m.

Glenoid labrum

Spinoglenoid notch (Inferior scapular notch)

Head of humerus

Glenoid process

Deltoid m.

Subdeltoid fascia

Infraspinatus m.

Glenoid labrum

Spinoglenoid notch

Glenohumeral joint capsule

Head of humerus

Articular cartilage

Glenoid process

Figure 4.12 Transverse view of the posterior aspect of the glenohumeral joint and glenoid labrum deep to the deltoid and infraspinatus muscles.

Acromion

Acromioclavicular (AC) ligament

Acromioclavicular (AC) joint

Distal clavicle

AC lig.

Acromion

AC joint

Distal clavicle

Figure 4.13 Coronal view of the acromioclavicular joint and ligament.

Arm

Muscles

Posterior Compartment

The main muscle of the posterior compartment of the arm is the triceps brachii. The triceps brachii is formed from 3 heads: the long head, the medial head, and the lateral head. The 3 heads join and form the triceps tendon, which crosses the elbow to insert on the olecranon process of the ulna.

Anterior Compartment

There are 3 muscles in the anterior compartment: coraco-brachialis, brachialis, and biceps brachii. Biceps brachii is superficial to coracobrachialis in the proximal half of the arm and superficial to brachialis in the distal half. The 2 heads of the biceps muscle (long and short) join and form the biceps tendon, which crosses the elbow through the antecubital fossa and inserts on the proximal radius. The tendon of brachialis crosses the elbow through the floor of the antecubital fossa to insert on the proximal ulna.

Nerves

Radial Nerve

The radial nerve begins in the axilla as the largest branch of the posterior cord of the brachial plexus. Along with the deep brachial artery, the nerve leaves the axilla and enters the posterior compartment of the arm by passing under the teres major muscle and between the long head of the triceps brachii and the medial aspect of the humerus. The nerve then courses diagonally in the radial groove of the humerus between the medial and lateral heads of the triceps brachii. In its course through the radial groove the nerve is first accompanied by the deep brachial artery and then by the radial collateral artery, a terminal branch of the deep brachial. While in the radial groove, the nerve gives off muscular branches to the triceps brachii muscle and 2 cutaneous branches, the inferior lateral cutaneous nerve of the arm and the posterior cutaneous nerve of the forearm. The spiral course of the radial groove brings the nerve across the posterior surface of the humerus to its lateral aspect, where the nerve leaves the groove and courses for a short distance between the lateral head of the triceps brachii and brachialis muscles. The nerve then pierces the lateral intermuscular septum to enter the anterior compartment near the position where the brachioradialis muscle begins to appear at its superior-most point of origin from the humerus. The brachioradialis muscle separates the nerve from the lateral head of the triceps brachii, and the nerve comes to lie for the remainder of its course in the fascial plane between the brachioradialis and brachialis muscles. The radial nerve crosses the elbow adjacent to the cubital fossa in this fascial plane and ends near the elbow joint by dividing into its terminal branches, the deep and superficial radial nerves.

Median Nerve

The median nerve arises in the axilla from its medial and lateral roots, branches of the medial and lateral cords of the brachial plexus. The nerve leaves the axilla along the anterior surface of the axillary artery and subsequently courses through the anterior compartment of the arm immediately adjacent to the brachial artery. In the distal half of the arm, the artery and nerve lie in a groove adjacent to the biceps brachii, brachialis, and medial head of triceps brachii muscles, with the nerve at the medial surface of the artery. The median nerve has no branches in the arm. The nerve crosses the elbow joint through the cubital fossa in the fascial plane between brachialis and pronator teres to course distally through the anterior compartment of the forearm.

Ulnar Nerve

The ulnar nerve arises in the axilla from the medial cord of the brachial plexus and leaves the axilla posteromedial to the axillary artery. For the first part of its course in the arm, the nerve lies posteromedial to the brachial artery in the anterior compartment. In the middle third of the arm, the nerve pierces the medial intermuscular septum and comes to lie along the medial surface of triceps brachii. The ulnar nerve has no branches in the arm. The nerve crosses the elbow joint posteriorly through the cubital tunnel near the ulnar groove of the medial epicondyle of the humerus to continue its course in the anterior compartment of the forearm.

Technique

Radial Nerve

MIDHUMERUS RADIAL NERVE
Transverse
FIG. 4.14

Begin with the patient in the supine position with the limb adducted, the elbow slightly flexed, and the forearm supinated. Position the probe transverse to the lateral aspect of the arm at about the midhumerus level. Direct the probe marker so that as you follow the nerve distally and the probe moves toward the anterior surface of the limb, the marker ends up directed toward the patient's right side (for the right limb, this means that initially, the probe marker should be directed posteriorly). Identify the hyperechoic cortex of the humerus, the triceps brachii muscle posteriorly, and the brachialis muscle at the anterolateral aspect of the humeral shaft. From this starting position, move the probe superiorly and inferiorly along the lateral aspect of the arm until you can identify the hyperechoic oval profile of the radial nerve as it emerges from the radial groove. The nerve becomes more readily visible as it moves away from the hyperechoic surface of the humerus into the fascial plane between the lateral head of triceps brachii and brachialis, accompanied by the radial collateral artery. The lateral intermuscular septum is seen as a thin hyperechoic fascial band between triceps brachii and brachialis.

PROXIMAL TO ELBOW JOINT RADIAL NERVE
Transverse
FIG. 4.15

Keeping the radial nerve centered in the image, continue scanning a short distance distally and observe that the brachioradialis muscle, as it takes origin from the lateral supracondylar ridge of the humerus, begins to appear between the lateral head of the triceps brachii and brachialis muscles. At this point, the radial nerve is separated from the lateral head of triceps brachii and comes to lie between the brachioradialis and brachialis muscles. One of the 2 cutaneous branches of the nerve that arise along its course in the radial groove,

Triceps brachii m. lateral head
Radial n.
Radial collateral a.
Brachialis m.
Diaphysis of humerus

Lateral intermuscular septum
Triceps brachii m. lateral head
Brachialis m.
Radial n.
Radial collateral a.
Diaphysis of humerus

Figure 4.14 Transverse view of the radial nerve in the plane between the lateral head of triceps brachii and brachialis muscles, accompanied by the radial collateral artery.

the posterior cutaneous nerve of the forearm, may commonly be seen (along with the radial collateral artery) as it diverges from the main trunk of the radial nerve near the brachioradialis muscle. As the brachioradialis muscle appears, the lateral head of triceps brachii and the posterior cutaneous nerve of the forearm end up on the superficial (posterolateral) aspect of the brachioradialis muscle, whereas the radial nerve and brachialis muscle end up on its deep (anteromedial) aspect. The radial nerve can be followed distally in the fascial plane between the brachioradialis and brachialis for the remainder of its course, until it ends by dividing into its terminal branches anterior to the elbow joint (see page 23 and 25).

Median and Ulnar Nerves

MIDHUMERUS
MEDIAN NERVE
ULNAR NERVE
Transverse
FIG. 4.16

The patient should be in the supine position with the arm abducted and externally rotated and the forearm supinated and slightly flexed. Position the probe transverse to the medial aspect of the arm a few centimeters distal to the midhumerus level, with the probe marker facing anteriorly. Identify the hyperechoic cortex of the humerus, biceps brachii, brachialis, and medial head of triceps brachii. Look for the pulsations of the brachial artery and identify the large hyperechoic median nerve at the medial surface of the artery. Identify the ulnar nerve 1 to 2 cm posterior to the brachial artery/median nerve, between the surface of the medial head of triceps and the overlying subcutaneous fat. In the subcutaneous fat between the positions of the median and ulnar nerves, the small hyperechoic medial cutaneous nerve of the forearm can usually be identified. By exerting the least pressure possible on the probe face while still maintaining good skin contact, the brachial veins alongside the brachial artery and the basilic vein in subcutaneous fat should become visible.

| **Figure 4.15** | Transverse view of the radial nerve in the fascial plane between the brachioradialis and brachialis muscles, a few centimeters proximal to the elbow joint. |

Labels in figure: Basilic v., Median n., Brachial a., Biceps brachii m., Brachialis m., Medial cutaneous nerve of forearm, Ulnar n., Triceps brachii m., Humerus

Lower ultrasound images labels: Medial cuteneous n. of forearm, Biceps m., Basilic v., Median n., Brachial a., Brachialis m., Ulnar n., Triceps m., Humerus

Figure 4.16 Transverse view of the median nerve alongside the brachial artery and the ulnar nerve at the superficial surface of triceps brachii muscle, just distal to the mid-humerus.

CLINICAL APPLICATIONS

These techniques can be used to guide a needle alongside the radial nerve for infiltration of a local anesthetic agent to produce a radial nerve block. Radial nerve blocks may be used in upper limb surgeries distal to the elbow (commonly as add-on regional anesthesia in addition to brachial plexus block), for postoperative pain control, or in the differential diagnosis of pain distal to the elbow. Ultrasound examination of the radial nerve may also be used for evaluation of possible nerve entrapment such as may occur in the presence of fractures involving the mid-diaphysis or lateral epicondyle of the humerus.

Ultrasound examination of the median and ulnar nerves in the arm is used for evaluation of possible nerve entrapment and compressive neuropathy in the distal half of the arm involving osteophytes and/or ligamentous bands. These techniques can also be used for needle guidance and infiltration of local anesthetic agents for regional anesthesia, although more distal sites (i.e., at the wrist) are more commonly utilized for median and ulnar blocks.

Elbow

Review of Anatomy

Elbow Joint

The elbow joint consists of 3 articulations between the humerus, radius, and ulna, all within a common joint capsule and synovial space. The articular surface of the humerus consists of the capitulum, which articulates with the head of the radius and the trochlea, which articulates with the trochlear notch of the ulna. The radial notch of the ulna articulates with the radial head. There are 2 anterior fossae on the humerus just above the articular surface: the radial fossa, which accommodates the radial head in flexion, and the coronoid fossa, which accommodates the coronoid process of the ulna in flexion. The olecranon fossa on the posterior surface of the humerus accommodates the olecranon process of the ulna in extension. Fat pads that separate the fibrous joint capsule from the synovial lining in these fossae are referred to clinically as the anterior fat pad (in the coronoid and radial fossae) and the posterior fat pad (in the olecranon fossa). The joint capsule is thickened to form the ulnar and radial collateral ligaments, and there is a thickened ring at the radial head, the annular ligament.

Muscles

The tendon of triceps brachii passes over the posterior fat pad and crosses the elbow joint to insert on the olecranon process of the ulna. Pronator teres and muscles arising from the common flexor tendon cross from the medial epicondyle to enter the anterior forearm compartment. Extensor muscles cross the elbow from the lateral epicondyle and supracondylar ridge to enter the posterior compartment of the forearm. The tendon of biceps brachii crosses the elbow joint through the cubital fossa to insert on the radial tuberosity. A tendinous sheet, the bicipital aponeurosis, extends from the medial side of the biceps tendon and attaches over the pronator teres muscle and proximal muscle mass of the common flexor tendon. The brachialis tendon crosses from the floor of the cubital fossa to insert on the ulnar tuberosity.

Cubital Fossa

The cubital fossa is a triangular depression at the anterior elbow formed by the brachioradialis muscle laterally, the pronator teres muscle medially, and a line interconnecting the humeral epicondyles superiorly. The brachialis muscle forms the bed of the fossa. Contents of the fossa include the biceps tendon, the brachial artery and accompanying veins, and the median nerve. The median cubital vein lies in the roof of the fossa, which is formed by skin and superficial fascia. The brachial artery normally bifurcates into the radial and ulnar arteries in the cubital fossa, although this division sometimes occurs more proximally in the axilla or arm.

Nerves

Radial Nerve

The radial nerve crosses the elbow joint just lateral to the cubital fossa in the fascial plane between brachioradialis and brachialis. The radial nerve continues distally, crossing anterior to the elbow joint at the part between the radius and the capitulum of the humerus where it divides into its terminal branches, the deep radial nerve and the superficial radial nerve. The deep radial nerve courses posteriorly and enters the substance of the supinator muscle, traveling between 2 layers of the muscle into the posterior compartment of the forearm, emerging as the posterior interosseous nerve. The superficial radial nerve joins the radial artery and continues distally in the anterior compartment under the brachioradialis muscle, winding across its distal tendon to supply the skin over the anatomical "snuffbox," dorsal aspect of the hand, thumb, and proximal index and middle fingers.

Median Nerve

The median nerve crosses the elbow joint through the cubital fossa in the fascial plane between brachialis and pronator teres, just medial to the brachial artery. The bicipital aponeurosis forms a protective layer over the contents of this fascial plane. The nerve enters the anterior compartment of the forearm by passing between the humeral and ulnar heads of pronator teres to continue its course in the forearm between the flexor digitorum superficialis and flexor digitorum profundus muscles and then crosses the wrist through the carpal tunnel into the hand.

Ulnar Nerve

The ulnar nerve leaves the posterior compartment of the arm by crossing the elbow joint posteriorly through the cubital tunnel near the ulnar groove of the medial epicondyle of the humerus. The arcuate ligament, which spans between the humeral and ulnar heads of flexor carpi ulnaris near their origins, forms the roof of the cubital tunnel, and the posterior layer of the ulnar collateral ligament of the elbow forms the floor (over the elbow joint capsule and ulnar groove of the humerus). The nerve enters the anterior compartment of the forearm between the 2 heads of flexor carpi ulnaris and courses through the forearm between flexor carpi ulnaris and flexor digitorum profundus and then crosses the wrist into the hand.

Technique

Cubital Fossa

**CUBITAL FOSSA
LATERAL CONTENTS**
Transverse
FIG. 4.17

The patient should be supine with the forearm supinated. A small pillow/bolster should be placed under the wrist to help maintain slight flexion at the elbow joint. Place the probe transversely over the elbow crease (probe marker toward the right) and adjust the position until you can clearly identify the hyperechoic profile of the capitulum and trochlea of the humerus. Identify the hyperechoic radial nerve in the fascial plane between the brachioradialis and brachialis muscles. The radial nerve typically divides into its deep and superficial branches near this position, giving it a bilobar appearance, and parts of one or both branches may appear hypoechoic because of anisotropy. Applying as little pressure as possible, identify the median cubital vein in the superficial fascia. Identify the biceps tendon at the surface of the brachialis muscle. The bicipital aponeurosis extends medially from the biceps tendon over the fascial plane between brachialis and pronator teres.

**CUBITAL FOSSA
MEDIAL CONTENTS**
Transverse
FIG. 4.18

Keeping the humeral trochlea in view, slide the probe medially until the pronator teres and the fascial plane between brachialis and pronator teres can be identified. In the superficial part of the fascial plane, locate the brachial artery and median nerve, and once again identify the bicipital aponeurosis bridging over the space between the 2 muscles.

Superficial and Deep Radial Nerves

**SUPERFICIAL RADIAL
NERVE
DEEP RADIAL NERVE**
Transverse
FIG. 4.19

Slide the probe laterally until the radial nerve is once again centered over the humeral capitulum. Slowly move the probe distally, following the radial nerve branches over the radial head and then over the supinator muscle surrounding the radial neck. With careful observation, the superficial and deep branches can be seen to diverge, with the deep radial

Figure 4.17 Transverse view of the lateral aspect of the cubital fossa and its contents. ECRB, extensor carpi radialis brevis; ECRL, extensor carpi radialis longus.

nerve moving laterally/deeply into the substance of the supinator muscle and the superficial radial nerve moving medially just under cover of the brachioradialis. Because of its oblique course, the deep radial nerve is more difficult to follow. The superficial radial nerve can be followed distally under the brachioradialis muscle until it moves alongside the radial artery.

Elbow Joint

ELBOW JOINT HUMEROULNAR COMPONENT
Longitudinal
FIG. 4.20

Slide the probe medially until it is centered over the humeral trochlea. Rotate the probe 90 degrees (marker directed superiorly) into the longitudinal axis of the humeroulnar joint. Adjust the position until the hyperechoic profile of the trochlea and coronoid fossa of the humerus and coronoid process of the ulna can be identified. The articular cartilage over the joint surfaces appears anechoic/hypoechoic. The fibrous joint capsule appears hyperechoic, and the anterior fat pad can be seen occupying the coronoid fossa inside the joint capsule. Identify the brachialis and pronator teres muscles overlying the joint.

ELBOW JOINT RADIOCAPITELLAR COMPONENT
Longitudinal
FIG. 4.21

Center the probe transversely over the capitulum and rotate the probe 90 degrees into the longitudinal axis of the radiocapitellar joint. Adjust the position until the profile of the capitulum of the humerus, the radial head, and proximal part of the radial neck can be identified. Identify the joint capsule and articular cartilage of the radiocapitellar joint. Locate the annular ligament, a thickening of the joint capsule ringing the head of the radius. The radial fossa can be seen just superior to the capitulum. The lateral aspect of the brachialis muscle can be seen overlying the joint and the supinator muscle surrounds the neck of the radius just over the distal attachment of the joint capsule.

Ulnar Nerve in the Cubital Tunnel

CUBITAL TUNNEL ULNAR NERVE
Transverse
FIG. 4.22

The patient should be supine with the arm abducted and externally rotated and the elbow slightly flexed. By palpation, identify the medial epicondyle of the humerus and the tip of the olecranon process of the

Figure 4.18 Transverse view of the medial aspect of the cubital fossa and its contents.

ulna. Place the probe across these bony landmarks with the marker side over the olecranon process. Identify the hyperechoic profile of the olecranon process, the humeroulnar joint space, and the ulnar groove and prominence of the medial epicondyle of the humerus. The ulnar nerve commonly appears as a hypoechoic/anechoic oval (because of anisotropy), but by tilting/fanning the probe its honeycomb appearance can usually be accentuated. Identify the hyperechoic band of arcuate ligament (aponeurosis of flexor carpi ulnaris) immediately superficial to the nerve spanning over and between the humeral and ulnar heads of flexor carpi ulnaris (you may need to slide the probe distally beyond the ulnar groove to visualize and identify the 2 heads of the muscle). Immediately deep to the nerve identify the hyperechoic fibrillar appearance of the posterior layer of the ulnar collateral ligament.

Keeping the nerve and the 2 heads of flexor carpi ulnaris in view, slide the probe distally a short distance beyond the cubital tunnel and observe as the 2 heads join together over the nerve (the hyperechoic honeycomb appearance of the nerve is more readily apparent in this position).

Triceps Brachii Muscle and Tendon

TRICEPS BRACHII MYOTENDINOUS JUNCTION
Longitudinal
FIG. 4.23

The patient should be seated alongside the examination table. The arm should be abducted and the elbow flexed to about 90 degrees, and the forearm fully pronated with the palm on the table surface (the "crab" position). Place the probe over the olecranon process and the distal triceps brachii muscle in the longitudinal axis of the arm (marker directed toward the shoulder). Adjust the probe position until the bony profile of the olecranon process of the ulna and the olecranon fossa of the humerus can be identified. The posterior fat

Extensor carpi radialis longus (ECRL) m. & Extensor carpi radialis brevis (ECRB) m.
Brachioradialis m.
Superficial radial n.
Deep radial n.
Tendon of biceps brachii
Supinator m.
Radius
Extensor carpi ulnaris m.
Extensor digitorum m.

Brachioradialis m.
Superficial radial n.
ECRL & ECRB
Deep radial n.
Supinator m.
Neck of radius

Figure 4.19 Transverse view of the superficial and deep branches of the radial nerve at the lateral aspect of the forearm just distal to the elbow joint.

pad can be seen in the olecranon fossa deep to the fibrous joint capsule. The distal triceps brachii muscle, myotendinous junction, and hyperechoic fibrillar triceps brachii tendon can be seen crossing over the olecranon fossa and joint space to the olecranon process.

TENDON OF TRICEPS BRACHII
Longitudinal
FIG. 4.24

Slide the probe distally along the triceps brachii tendon until the tapering beak of the tendon insertion onto the olecranon process can be identified.

Common Flexor Tendon and Ulnar Collateral Ligament

COMMON FLEXOR TENDON
ULNAR COLLATERAL LIGAMENT
Longitudinal
FIG. 4.25

The patient should be supine with the arm abducted and externally rotated and the elbow flexed to approximately 90 degrees. Place the marker end of the probe over the anterior surface of the medial epicondyle along the longitudinal

axis of the forearm. The probe should be tilted so that the ultrasound beam is directed from anterior to posterior (not across the elbow from medial to lateral). Adjust the position and tilt until the prominence of the medial epicondyle, the concavity between the epicondyle and the margin of the trochlea, the humeroulnar joint space, and the margin of the trochlear notch of the ulna can be seen. Identify the normally short hyperechoic common flexor tendon and the myotendinous junction of the common flexor muscle mass. The anterior layer of the ulnar collateral ligament can be seen spanning the joint space immediately deep to the common flexor tendon and muscle.

Common Extensor Tendon and Radial Collateral Ligament

COMMON EXTENSOR TENDON
RADIAL COLLATERAL LIGAMENT
FIG. 4.26

The patient should be supine with the arm adducted, the elbow slightly flexed, and the forearm in mid-pronation with the ulnar border of the hand resting on the upper thigh. Position the probe

Brachialis m.
Trochlea
Anterior fat pad
Coronoid fossa
Humerus
Pronator teres m.
Joint capsule
Articular cartilage of humeroulnar joint
Coronoid process
Ulna

Pronator teres m.
Brachialis m.
Joint capsule
Anterior fat pad
Trochlea
Coronoid process of ulna
Coronoid fossa
Humerus
Articular cartilage of humeroulnar joint

Figure 4.20 Longitudinal view of the humeroulnar component of the elbow joint.

along the longitudinal axis of the forearm with the marker end of the probe over the lateral epicondyle. Adjust the probe position until the hyperechoic profile of the lateral epicondyle of the humerus and the head of the radius can be identified. Locate the tapering beak of the common extensor origin from the lateral epicondyle and identify the annular ligament at the radial head (tilting/fanning the probe as needed to accentuate its echogenicity). Identify the radial collateral ligament at the deep surface of the common extensor tendon, spanning from the slight concavity along lateral epicondyle across the radiocapitellar joint and fusing with the annular ligament.

CLINICAL APPLICATIONS

These techniques can be used to guide needles alongside the radial, median, or ulnar nerves for infiltration of local anesthetic agents to produce nerve blocks. Radial nerve blocks may be used in upper limb surgeries distal to the elbow (commonly as add-on regional anesthesia in addition to brachial plexus block), for postoperative pain control, or in the differential diagnosis of pain distal to the elbow. With ultrasound guidance, the median nerve can be blocked in the cubital fossa alongside the brachial artery and accompanying veins. Ulnar nerve blocks at the elbow should be proximal to the cubital tunnel to avoid possible nerve compression resulting from injection of anesthetic fluid around the nerve within the relatively limited space of the tunnel. The forearm and wrist are more common sites for median and ulnar blocks.

Ultrasound examination of these nerves may also be used for evaluation of possible nerve entrapment. The posterior interosseous branch nerve can be entrapped in its course through the supinator muscle. The median nerve can be entrapped in its course between the heads of pronator teres, and the cubital tunnel is a common site of ulnar nerve entrapment and compression. The ulnar nerve can also subluxate/dislocate from the cubital tunnel over the anterior surface of the medial epicondyle with flexion/extension.

Ultrasound examination can be used for cannulating veins (e.g., median cubital, cephalic, and basilic) and for evaluation of brachial artery aneurysm or stenosis.

Ultrasound examination can be used for evaluation of possible biceps, common flexor, or common extensor tendonitis/tendinosis or ligamentous strains and tears (e.g., ulnar collateral and radial collateral ligaments of the elbow). The anterior and posterior fat pads are displaced from their fossae when fluid accumulates within the joint space (joint effusion or bleeding into the joint space in the presence of intra-articular fractures), and these techniques can be used for needle guidance into the elbow joint space for aspiration or injection.

Biceps brachii m.
Brachialis m.
Capitulum
Fat pad
Radial fossa
Articular cartilage of radiocapitellar joint

Brachioradialis m.
Supinator m.
Neck of radius
Head of radius
Joint capsule and anular ligament

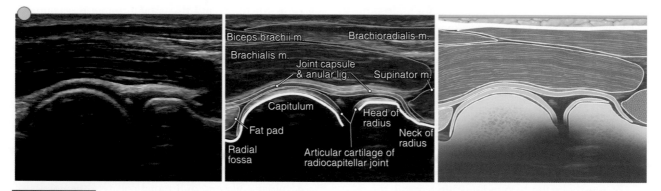

Biceps brachii m.
Brachialis m.
Joint capsule & anular lig.
Capitulum
Fat pad
Radial fossa
Articular cartilage of radiocapitellar joint
Brachioradialis m.
Supinator m.
Head of radius
Neck of radius

Figure 4.21   Longitudinal view of the radiocapitellar component of the elbow joint.

Aponeurosis of flexor carpi ulnaris (arcuate ligament)
Ulnar n.
Posterior band of ulnar collateral ligament
Humeroulnar joint
Trochlea
Olecranon

Flexor carpi ulnaris m. ulnar head
Arcuate ligament
Flexor carpi ulnaris m. humeral head
Ulnar n.
Olecranon process of ulna
Humeroulnar joint
Posterior band of ulnar collateral ligament
Medial epicondyle
Ulnar groove

Figure 4.22   Transverse view of the ulnar nerve in the cubital tunnel.

Figure 4.23 Longitudinal view of the triceps brachii muscle, myotendinous junction, and tendon at the posterior aspect of the elbow joint.

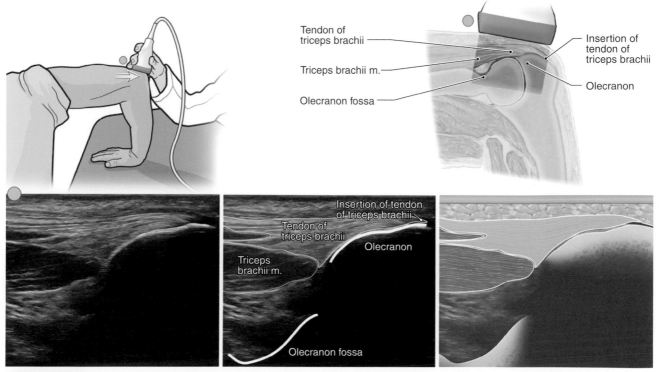

Figure 4.24 Longitudinal view of the tendon of triceps brachii inserting onto the olecranon process of the ulna.

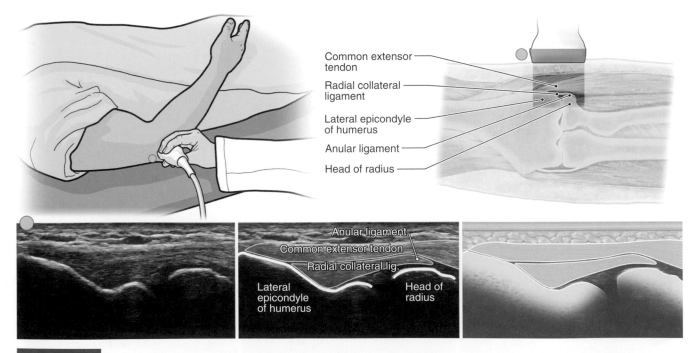

Figure 4.25 Longitudinal view of the anterior layer of the ulnar collateral ligament and overlying common flexor tendon.

Figure 4.26 Longitudinal view of the radial collateral ligament and overlying common extensor tendon.

Distal Forearm, Wrist, and Hand

Review of the Anatomy

Anterior Compartment Tendons and Carpal Tunnel

The muscles of the anterior compartment of the forearm include the flexors of the wrist, the superficial and deep digital flexors, flexor pollicis longus, and the 2 pronators of the forearm. The tendons of flexor digitorum superficialis, flexor digitorum profundus, and flexor pollicis longus enter the hand through the carpal tunnel, along with the median nerve. The floor and sides of the tunnel are formed by the arch of proximal and distal rows of carpal bones (and associated radiocarpal, ulnocarpal, and palmar intercarpal ligaments), and the roof is formed by the transverse carpal ligament (flexor retinaculum), which attaches medially to the pisiform and hamate bones and laterally to the tubercles of the scaphoid and trapezium. The tendon of flexor carpi radialis crosses into the hand along the medial surface of the scaphoid just outside the carpal tunnel, between 2 layers of the transverse carpal ligament.

Median Nerve

The median nerve travels through the anterior compartment of the forearm in the plane between flexor digitorum superficialis and flexor digitorum profundus. The median nerve and its anterior interosseous branch innervate most of the muscles of the anterior forearm (except the medial half of flexor digitorum superficialis and flexor carpi ulnaris, which are supplied by the ulnar nerve). At the wrist, the median nerve moves superficially between the tendon of flexor carpi radialis and the tendons of flexor digitorum superficialis and crosses into the hand through the carpal tunnel (along with the tendons of the digital flexor muscles) just under cover of the transverse carpal ligament.

Ulnar Nerve

The ulnar nerve enters the anterior compartment of the forearm between the 2 heads of flexor carpi ulnaris and courses through the forearm between flexor carpi ulnaris and flexor digitorum profundus. In the forearm, the ulnar nerve supplies motor innervation to flexor carpi ulnaris and the ulnar half of flexor digitorum profundus. The ulnar nerve, accompanied by the ulnar artery, crosses the wrist through Guyon's canal, between the pisiform bone and the hook of the hamate bone. The roof of Guyon's canal is the palmar carpal ligament (a thickened region of deep forearm fascia), and the floor is the transverse carpal ligament.

Radial and Ulnar Arteries

The brachial artery divides into its terminal branches, the radial and ulnar arteries, in the cubital fossa. The radial artery, accompanied by the superficial radial nerve, crosses superficially to the pronator teres tendon, first lying just under cover of the brachioradialis muscle/tendon and then lateral to the tendon of flexor carpi radialis in the distal forearm. The ulnar artery passes deep to the pronator teres muscle and joins the ulnar nerve between flexor carpi ulnaris and flexor digitorum profundus for the remainder of its course in the forearm and then through Guyon's canal into the hand.

Posterior Compartment Tendons and Extensor Retinaculum

The muscles of the posterior compartment of the forearm include brachioradialis, supinator, extensors of the wrist and digits, abductor pollicis longus, extensors pollicis longus and brevis, and extensor indicis. The muscles of the posterior compartment are innervated by the radial nerve or its deep branch/posterior interosseous nerve. The tendons of wrist and digital extensors, and abductor pollicis longus, cross into the hand through 6 compartments formed by the extensor retinaculum related to the lateral surface of the radius, the dorsal surface of the radius, and the medial surface of the ulna. Just distal to the extensor retinaculum, the tendon of extensor pollicis longus forms the medial/posterior boundary of the anatomical snuffbox, and the tendons of extensor pollicis brevis and abductor pollicis longus form its lateral/anterior boundary. The floor of the snuffbox is formed by the scaphoid and trapezium, and its roof is formed by skin and superficial fascia. The radial artery curves dorsally from the anterior forearm compartment through the snuffbox into the hand, and branches of the superficial radial nerve and the cephalic vein course through the superficial fascia of the snuffbox roof.

63

Intrinsic Muscles of the Hand

The intrinsic muscles of the hand include the palmar and dorsal interosseous muscles, 4 lumbrical muscles, adductor pollicis, 3 hypothenar muscles, and the 3 thenar muscles: abductor pollicis brevis, flexor pollicis brevis, and opponens pollicis. The largest of the thenar muscles, opponens pollicis, originates from the tubercles of the scaphoid and trapezium and the adjacent palmar surface of the flexor retinaculum and wraps over the first metacarpal to insert along its lateral surface. The opponens lies deep to the 2 smaller thenar muscles. The tendon of flexor pollicis longus leaves the carpal tunnel and passes between the adductor pollicis muscle and the thenar muscles to reach its fibrous tunnel. Emerging from the carpal tunnel, the median nerve divides into its terminal branches, the recurrent branch to the thenar muscles, small motor branches for the first and second lumbrical muscles, and common palmar digital branches for the radial 3½ digits. Just distal to the pisiform bone, the ulnar nerve divides into its terminal branches, the superficial (palmar cutaneous) branch and the deep (motor) branch. The ulnar nerve innervates all of the intrinsic hand muscles except the thenar muscles and the first and second lumbricals, which are supplied by the median nerve, and provides common dorsal digital branches (via the dorsal cutaneous branch, which leaves the nerve proximal to the wrist) and common palmar digital branches to the ring and little fingers.

Digits and Digital Flexor Tendons

Each digit is associated with a metacarpal bone and a proximal, middle, and distal phalanx (the thumb only has a proximal and a distal phalanx). The joints of the digits are the metacarpophalangeal (head of metacarpal and base of proximal phalanx), proximal interphalangeal (head of proximal phalanx and base of middle phalanx), and distal interphalangeal (head of middle phalanx and base of distal phalanx). After emerging from the carpal tunnel, the flexor tendons of the digits cross the palm and enter fibrous sheaths, which begin just proximal to the metacarpophalangeal joints, for their course along the palmar surfaces of the digits. The fibrous sheaths are made up by 5 annular pulleys (short fibrous canals or arches) and intervening X-shaped (cruciate) ligaments, which are attached to palmar plates (palmar ligaments) of the metacarpophalangeal joints and the palmar surfaces of the phalanges. Palmar plates (ligaments) are wedgelike fibrocartilaginous ligaments that reinforce the joint capsules of the metacarpophalangeal and interphalangeal joints.

Technique

Distal Forearm

**DISTAL FOREARM
MEDIAN NERVE**
Transverse
FIG. 4.27

The patient should be supine with the arm slightly abducted, the forearm supinated, and the limb resting on the examination table. Place the probe transversely over the anterior surface between the middle and distal thirds of the forearm and identify the hyperechoic profiles and acoustic shadows of the radius and ulna. Adjust the probe position and tilt/fan the probe until the hyperechoic honeycomb appearance of the median nerve can be identified. The nerve is in the plane between flexor digitorum superficialis and flexor digitorum profundus, and flexor pollicis longus is just lateral to the nerve. Identify the myotendinous junction/tendon of flexor carpi radialis at the superficial surface of flexor digitorum superficialis. Just lateral to the tendon of flexor carpi radialis identify the radial artery. The superficial radial nerve is seen immediately lateral to the radial artery. Slide the probe distally a short distance until the pronator quadratus muscle can be identified crossing between the ulna and radius.

**DISTAL FOREARM
ULNAR NERVE
ULNAR ARTERY**
Transverse
FIG. 4.28

Place the probe transversely over the anterior surface just beyond the middle of the forearm and once again identify flexor digitorum superficialis and flexor digitorum profundus. Slide the probe medially until the flexor carpi ulnaris muscle appears at the medial border of the anterior compartment, medial to the digital flexor muscles. Identify the ulnar nerve and artery in the plane between flexor carpi ulnaris and flexor digitorum profundus and just deep to flexor digitorum superficialis.

Flexor carpi radialis (FCR) m.

Radial a.

Superficial radial n.

Flexor pollicis longus (FPL) m.

Radius

Flexor digitorum superficialis (FDS) m.

Median n.

Flexor digitorum profundus (FDP) m.

Ulna

Radial a.

FCR

FDS

Superficial radial n.

Median n.

FPL

FDP

Radius

Proximal fibers of pronator quadratus m.

Ulna

Figure 4.27 Transverse view of the median nerve in the distal forearm, in the plane between flexor digitorum superficialis (FDS) and flexor digitorum profundus (FDP). FCR, flexor carpi radialis; FPL, flexor pollicis longus.

65

Wrist: Carpal Tunnel and Guyon's Canal

**CARPAL TUNNEL
MEDIAN NERVE**
Transverse
FIG. 4.29

The patient should be supine with the forearm supinated and the back of the wrist resting on a small pillow/bolster. Place the probe transversely over the distal wrist crease and adjust the position until the hyperechoic profiles of the scaphoid tubercle and pisiform bone can be identified at the lateral and medial borders of the carpal tunnel. Carefully tilting/fanning the probe, identify the hyperechoic reflection of the transverse carpal ligament (flexor retinaculum) and the digital flexor tendons. Owing to anisotropy, the appearance of the ligament and tendons changes dramatically with small changes in tilt of the probe face. The median nerve usually appears as a hypoechoic oval structure just deep to the transverse carpal ligament (flexor retinaculum). The honeycomb appearance of the nerve can usually be accentuated by careful tilting/fanning of the probe (again because of anisotropy). The tendon of flexor pollicis longus is usually located immediately deep/

lateral to the median nerve but is sometimes difficult to see because of anisotropy. Slide the probe proximally, keeping the nerve in view, and follow the nerve back out of the carpal tunnel into the distal forearm between the digital flexor muscles and their tendons/myotendinous junctions. Return the probe to the position between the scaphoid tubercle and pisiform bone. Remembering the effects of anisotropy on tendon appearance, identify the tendon of flexor carpi radialis in a shallow groove along the medial aspect of the scaphoid tubercle, just outside the carpal tunnel. Just lateral to the pisiform bone, identify the pulsating ulnar artery with the ulnar nerve on its medial side, as they cross over the flexor retinaculum through Guyon's canal. Note the hyperechoic fibers of the palmar carpal ligament roofing over the artery and nerve in this position.

**GUYON'S CANAL
ULNAR NERVE
ULNAR ARTERY**
Transverse
FIG. 4.30

Slide the probe medially, bringing the ulnar artery and nerve in Guyon's canal closer to the center of the image. Carefully tilting/fanning the probe, again identify the ulnar nerve and artery along

Figure 4.28 Transverse view of the ulnar artery and nerve in the plane between flexor digitorum profundus and flexor carpi ulnaris.

with the roof (palmar carpal ligament) and floor (flexor retinaculum) of the canal. The nerve can often be seen dividing into its superficial and deep branches just distal to the pisiform bone.

Wrist: Extensor Retinaculum Compartments

COMPARTMENTS 3, 4, AND 5
TENDON OF EXTENSOR POLLICIS LONGUS
TENDON OF EXTENSOR DIGITORUM
TENDON OF EXTENSOR INDICIS
TENDON OF EXTENSOR DIGITI MINIMI
Transverse
FIG. 4.31

The patient should be supine with the forearm pronated and the forearm and palm resting on the examination table. Place the probe transversely over the dorsum of the wrist with the non-marker side of the probe over the prominence of the head of the ulna. Identify the head of the ulna and the expanded distal end of the radius. Slide back and forth over this position until you can identify the small prominence on the dorsal surface of the radius, the dorsal radial tubercle. Identify the tendon of extensor pollicis longus in extensor compartment 3 at the medial surface of the dorsal radial tubercle (often in a shallow bony groove). Medial to compartment 3, identify the large compartment 4 containing the tendons of extensor digitorum and extensor indicis. Just medial to compartment 4, over the radial side of the head of the ulna, identify

the tendon of extensor digiti minimi in compartment 5. Carefully tilting/fanning the probe, identify the hyperechoic extensor retinaculum and its fibrous bands separating the compartments.

COMPARTMENT 6
TENDON OF EXTENSOR CARPI ULNARIS
Transverse
FIG. 4.32

Slide the probe medially onto the ulnar side of the wrist. Adjust the probe position until it is centered over the rounded prominence of the ulnar head and the base of the ulnar styloid process. The tendon of extensor carpi ulnaris is located in compartment 6, in the groove between the ulnar head and base of the styloid process. Because of the narrow bony surface at the side of the wrist, it is not possible to maintain skin contact all the way across the probe face.

COMPARTMENT 2
TENDON OF EXTENSOR CARPI RADIALIS LONGUS
TENDON OF EXTENSOR CARPI RADIALIS BREVIS
FIG. 4.33

Slide the probe back laterally across the dorsum of the wrist and again identify the dorsal radial tubercle. Continue laterally just beyond the tubercle onto the posterolateral surface of the radius (where again it is impossible to maintain skin contact across the entire probe face). In compartment 2, identify the tendons of extensor carpi radialis brevis and extensor carpi radialis longus. The tendon of extensor carpi radialis

Flexor retinaculum (transverse carpal ligament)
Median n.
Palmar carpal ligament
Ulnar a. & n. in Guyon's canal
Tendon of flexor carpi radialis (FCR)
Pisiform
Scaphoid
Tendon of flexor pollicis longus (FPL)
Tendons of flexor digitorum superficialis (FDS) & profundus (FDP)

*Visibility of tendons in carpal tunnel are variably echoic due to anisotropy.

Thenar m.
Flexor retinaculum
Palmar carpal lig.
FCR
Scaphoid tubercle
FPL*
Pisiform
Median n.
Ulnar a. & n.
FDS &FDP*

Figure 4.29 Transverse view of the median nerve in the carpal tunnel along with the tendons of flexor digitorum superficialis (FDS), flexor digitorum profundus (FDP), and flexor pollicis longus (FPL). The tendon of flexor carpi radialis (FCR) is just outside the carpal tunnel.

brevis is alongside the lateral surface of the dorsal radial tubercle. Slide the probe distally and observe the tendon of extensor pollicis longus as it moves laterally across the radial carpal extensor tendons.

**COMPARTMENT 1
TENDON OF EXTENSOR
    POLLICIS BREVIS
TENDON OF ABDUCTOR
    POLLICIS LONGUS
FIG. 4.34**

Return the probe to the view of the radial carpal extensor tendons in compartment 2, and slide the probe further laterally/anteriorly onto the narrow lateral surface of the radius, at the base of the radial styloid process. Identify the tendons of extensor pollicis brevis and abductor pollicis longus in compartment 1. These tendons are often separated by a dense fibrous band spanning the compartment. Look for the cephalic vein and branches of the superficial radial nerve near compartment 1 in this position (which is just proximal to the anatomical snuffbox).

Hand: Thenar Eminence

**THENAR MUSCLES
TENDON OF FLEXOR
    POLLICIS LONGUS
ADDUCTOR POLLICIS
FIRST DORSAL
    INTEROSSEOUS
    MUSCLE
Transverse
FIG. 4.35**

The patient should be supine with the forearm fully supinated and the dorsum of the hand resting on the examination table. Place the probe over the middle of the thenar eminence, transverse to the long axis of the first metacarpal bone. Adjust the probe position until the first and second metacarpal bones can be identified. The scan depth should be adjusted until the bright skin/air interface can be seen at the dorsum of the hand. The hyperechoic tendon of flexor pollicis longus is easily seen passing over the palmar surface of adductor pollicis, between adductor pollicis and the thenar muscles. Identify the adductor pollicis muscle, the first dorsal interosseous muscle lying posterior to it, and the thenar muscles. The thenar muscles can be difficult to identify definitively, but the abductor pollicis brevis tends to be the most superficial of

 Figure 4.30 Transverse view of the ulnar artery and nerve in Guyon's canal. FDP, flexor digitorum profundus; FDS, flexor digitorum superficialis.

the 3 over most of the thenar eminence. By sliding the probe proximally and distally, the inserting fibers of opponens pollicis can be seen as they curve over the first metacarpal along its lateral margin. By sliding the probe distally and slightly medially, the hypoechoic oval profile of the first lumbrical muscle can be identified as it takes origin from the flexor digitorum profundus tendon of the index finger.

Hand: Flexor Tendons of the Digits

METACARPOPHALANGEAL JOINT
FLEXOR TENDONS OF THE DIGITS
Longitudinal
FIG. 4.36

The patient should be supine with the forearm supinated, the digits adducted and extended, and the dorsum of the hand resting on the examination table. Place the probe along the longitudinal axis of a digit over the location of the metacarpophalangeal joint. Adjust the probe position until the head of the metacarpal, the metacarpophalangeal joint, and the base of the proximal phalanx are near the center of the image. Identify the flexor tendons overlying the bones and joint, and carefully adjust the probe orientation until the hyperechoic fibrillar appearance of the tendons can be seen throughout the

image. Look for the area proximal to the metacarpal head where the tendons of flexor digitorum superficialis and flexor digitorum profundus converge near their entry into the fibrous digital sheath. At the metacarpal head and for some distance proximally, the tendons are separated from the surface of the metacarpal bone by the hyperechoic palmar plate (palmar metacarpal ligament) reinforcing the joint capsule. The palmar ligament (palmar plate) of the metacarpophalangeal joint is attached along the base of the proximal phalanx and tapers proximally, blending with the metacarpophalangeal joint capsule. Immediately superficial to the tendons, at the metacarpal head, attempt to identify the first annular (A1) pulley, by carefully sliding/tilting/fanning the probe while centered over the metacarpal head. In their long axis, normal pulleys are seen as relatively thin anechoic/hypoechoic bands with thin hyperechoic margins on both sides.

METACARPOPHALANGEAL JOINT
FLEXOR TENDONS OF THE DIGITS
Transverse
FIG. 4.37

Centered over the metacarpal head, rotate the probe 90 degrees into the transverse axis. Identify the hyperechoic profile of the metacarpal head, the palmar plate, and the flexor

 Transverse view of extensor retinaculum compartments 3, 4, and 5. Compartment 3 contains the tendon of extensor pollicis longus (EPL). Compartment 4 contains the tendons of extensor digitorum and extensor indicis. Compartment 5 contains the tendon of extensor digiti minimi.

tendons within their fibrous sheath. The first annular (A1) pulley is seen as a thin anechoic horseshoe-shaped band arching over the flexor tendons and attaching along the sides of the palmar plate. Look for the pulsations of palmar digital arteries and hyperechoic digital nerves on either side of the fibrous tendon sheath.

to be slightly thicker distally than it is at its proximal edge. Notice that the fibrillar appearance and direction of the tendon fibers change distally as the superficialis tendon separates into bands that insert on the middle phalanx and allow the profundus tendon to continue on to the distal phalanx.

PROXIMAL PHALANX FLEXOR TENDONS OF THE DIGITS
Longitudinal
FIG. 4.38

Rotate the probe back into the longitudinal axis over the metacarpophalangeal joint, and keeping the tendons and proximal phalanx in view, slide the probe a short distance distally until the central part of the palmar surface of the proximal phalanx is near the center of the image. Immediately superficial to the flexor tendons, look for the "bright-dark-bright" appearance of the second annular (A2) pulley, which is typically much easier to identify in its longitudinal axis than is the first annular pulley. The second annular pulley tends

PROXIMAL PHALANX FLEXOR TENDONS OF THE DIGITS
Transverse
FIG. 4.39

Centered over the second annular (A2) pulley, rotate the probe 90 degrees into the transverse axis of the digit. Identify the diaphysis of the proximal phalanx, the flexor tendons in their fibrous sheath, and the second annular pulley. The pulley appears as a thin anechoic horseshoe-shaped band (with occasional internal echoes) arching over the flexor tendons and attaching along the margins of the anterior surface of the proximal phalanx. Look for the proper palmar digital neurovascular bundles on either side of the fibro-osseous tendon tunnel.

Extensor retinaculum

Head of ulna

Tendon of extensor carpi ulnaris

Styloid process of ulna

Extensor retinaculum

Head of ulna

Base of styloid process of ulna

Extensor carpi ulnaris

Figure 4.32 Transverse view of the tendon of extensor carpi ulnaris in compartment 6 of the extensor retinaculum.

Figure 4.33 Transverse view of the tendons of extensor carpi radialis longus (ECRL) and extensor carpi radialis brevis (ECRB) in compartment 2 of the extensor retinaculum. EPL, extensor pollicis longus.

Figure 4.34 Transverse view of the tendons of extensor pollicis brevis (EPB) and abductor pollicis longus (APL) in compartment 1 of the extensor retinaculum.

Abductor
pollicis brevis m.

Opponens
pollicis m.

Flexor pollicis brevis m.

Tendon of flexor
pollicis longus (FPL)

1st lumbrical m.

1st
metacarpal

1st dorsal
interosseous m.

2nd
metacarpal

Adductor
pollicis m.

Abductor pollicis
brevis m.

1st lumbrical m.

Flexor pollicis
brevis m.

Opponens
pollicis m.

FPL

Adductor
pollicis m.

1st metacarpal

1st dorsal
interosseous m.

2nd
metacarpal

Figure 4.35 Transverse view of the thenar muscles, the tendon of flexor pollicis longus, adductor pollicis, and the first dorsal interosseous muscle.

Tendon of flexor digitorum superficialis
Tendon of flexor digitorum profundus
A1 pulley
Proximal phalanx
Palmar plate (ligament)
Metacarpophalangeal (MCP) joint

A1 pulley
Tendon of flexor digitorum superficialis
Tendon of flexor digitorum profundus
Palmar plate (ligament)
Base of proximal phalanx
Head of metacarpal
MCP joint

Figure 4.36 Longitudinal view of the tendons of flexor digitorum superficialis and flexor digitorum profundus at the metacarpophalangeal (MCP) joint, along with the palmar ligament of the joint and the first annular (A1) pulley of the fibrous tendon sheath.

A1 pulley

Tendons of flexor digitorum superficialis (FDS) & profundus (FDP)

Palmar digital neurovascular bundle (NVB)

Palmar plate (ligament)

Head of metacarpal

A1 pulley

Palmar digital NVB

FDS & FDP

Palmar plate (ligament)

Palmar digital NVB

Head of metacarpal

Figure 4.37 Transverse view of the tendons of flexor digitorum superficialis (FDS) and flexor digitorum profundus (FDP) over the head of the metacarpal bone, along with the palmar ligament of the metacarpophalangeal joint and the first annular (A1) pulley of the fibrous tendon sheath. NVB, neurovascular bundle.

Palmar plate (ligament) of PIP joint

Proximal interphalangeal (PIP) joint

Proximal phalanx

Joint capsule

Tendon of flexor digitorum superficialis (FDS)

A2 pulley

Tendon of flexor digitorum profundus (FDP)

A2 pulley

Palmar plate (ligament) of PIP joint

FDS

FDP

Diaphysis of proximal phalanx

Joint capsule & extracapsular fibrofatty tissue

Head of proximal phalanx

Figure 4.38 Longitudinal view of the tendons of flexor digitorum superficialis (FDS) and flexor digitorum profundus (FDP) over the diaphysis of the proximal phalanx, along with second annular (A2) pulley of the fibrous tendon sheath. PIP, proximal interphalangeal.

Figure 4.39 Transverse view of the tendons of flexor digitorum superficialis (FDS) and flexor digitorum profundus (FDP) over the diaphysis of the proximal phalanx, along with second annular (A2) pulley of the fibrous tendon sheath. NVB, neurovascular bundle.

Labels on figure:
- Palmar digital NVB
- A2 pulley
- Diaphysis of proximal phalanx
- Tendons of flexor digitorum superficialis (FDS) & profundus (FDP)
- Palmar digital NVB
- A2 pulley
- Palmar digital NVB
- FDS & FDP
- Diaphysis of proximal phalanx

CLINICAL APPLICATIONS

These techniques can be used to guide needles into position to inject local anesthetic agents along the median and ulnar nerves in the distal forearm or wrist to produce regional anesthesia for surgical procedures in the hand. Ultrasound examination is also used for evaluation of potential nerve compression injuries such as the median nerve in the carpal tunnel or the ulnar nerve in Guyon's canal.

Ultrasound examination is being increasingly used in the evaluation and treatment of a variety of muscular,

tendinous, and ligamentous strains/tears or other dysfunctions. For example, the first extensor compartment is involved in De Quervain's tenosynovitis, which causes pain and dysfunction of abductor pollicis longus and extensor pollicis brevis. Nodularity and/or thickening of the first annular pulley is often associated with "trigger-finger," and the other annular pulleys (especially the second and fourth) may be torn or ruptured in rock-climbing injuries.

5

Lower Limb

Proximal Thigh and Inguinal Region

Review of the Anatomy

Bones

The bones of the proximal thigh and groin are those of the pelvis and femur.

Pelvic Bones

The pelvic bones (os coxae) are formed by the fusion of the ilium, ischium, and pubis. The expanded upper part of the ilium, the wing (ala), has an anterior surface that forms part of the posterior abdominal wall and a posterior surface that is part of the gluteal region. The iliac crest is superior to the ala and extends from the anterior superior iliac spine (ASIS) anteriorly to the posterior superior iliac spine posteriorly. The anterior inferior iliac spine projects from the anterior edge of the ilium a few centimeters inferior and medial to the ASIS just above the lateral aspect of the socket of the hip joint, the acetabulum. The acetabulum is located laterally on the pelvic bone where the 3 bones come together, just inferior to the approximate midpoint of the inguinal ligament.

Femur

The head of the femur articulates with the acetabulum of the pelvic bone to form the hip joint. The head of the femur is attached to the body of the femur by the neck of the femur, which projects inferolaterally (and slightly anteriorly) from the head of the femur to the proximal part of the body of the femur, at an angle between 120 and 135 degrees in the frontal plane. The greater and lesser trochanters and intertrochanteric areas are adjacent to the junction between the neck and body of the femur. The large greater trochanter projects superiorly from the lateral aspect of this junction and has a depression, the trochanteric fossa, along its posteromedial surface. The lesser trochanter projects posteromedially from the body of the femur just below the junction between the neck and body. The greater and lesser trochanters are connected posteriorly by a prominent bony ridge, the intertrochanteric crest. Anteriorly, the trochanters are connected by a small bony ridge, the intertrochanteric line.

Hip Joint Capsule

The fibrous capsule of the hip joint attaches along the acetabular margin proximally and the intertrochanteric line and femoral neck adjacent to the intertrochanteric fossa. A synovial membrane attaches along the margins of the articular surfaces of the acetabulum and femoral head and descends along the neck of the femur before reflecting to line the interior of the fibrous membrane. The fibrous membrane is reinforced by 3 thickenings: the iliofemoral, pubofemoral, and ischiofemoral ligaments. The iliofemoral ligament is attached to the margin of the acetabulum proximally and the intertrochanteric line distally, reinforcing the joint capsule anteriorly. Although the hip joint is inherently much more stable than the glenohumeral joint, the bony rim of the acetabulum is additionally elevated by a fibrocartilaginous acetabular labrum.

Muscles

The muscles of the thigh are divided into 3 compartments by the fascia lata and its intermuscular septae. In addition, iliacus and psoas major enter the thigh from the posterior abdominal wall and insert through a common tendon (iliopsoas) onto the lesser trochanter of the femur. The anterior compartment muscles include sartorius and quadriceps femoris. The medial compartment muscles are pectineus, adductor brevis, adductor longus, adductor magnus, gracilis, and obturator externus. The posterior compartment muscles are the hamstrings: biceps femoris, semitendinosus, and semimembranosus.

With respect to muscular anatomy, this section focuses on a small subset of muscles in the proximal-most part of the thigh related to the ASIS, femoral triangle, and hip joint, plus a brief overview of the medial compartment muscles in the proximal thigh. The anterior and posterior compartments are discussed in additional detail in subsequent sections.

Iliacus and Psoas Major

Iliacus originates from the anterior abdominal surface (iliac fossa) of the pelvic bone. The psoas major muscle originates from transverse processes and adjacent bodies of the lumbar vertebrae. The 2 muscles enter the thigh inferior to the inguinal ligament and form the lateral half of the floor of the femoral triangle, passing over the hip joint and medial aspect of the neck of the femur to insert through a common tendon (iliopsoas tendon) onto the lesser trochanter of the femur.

Sartorius

Sartorius originates from the medial aspect of the ASIS, crosses the thigh from lateral to medial and inserts along with gracilis and semitendinosus on the medial aspect of the proximal tibia.

Tensor Fasciae Latae

The tensor fasciae latae muscle originates along a line that begins at the lateral aspect of the ASIS and extends a few centimeters posteriorly along the iliac crest as far as the tubercle of the crest, and inserts via the iliotibial tract, a thickened band of the fascia lata, onto the proximal tibia.

Gluteus Medius and Minimus

The gluteus medius and minimus muscles originate from the gluteal surface of the iliac ala nearly as far anteriorly as the ASIS and so come partially into view in ultrasound (US) images of proximal thigh muscles near the ASIS.

Rectus Femoris

The rectus femoris muscle originates mainly from the anterior inferior iliac spine (a few centimeters inferomedial to the ASIS) and inserts along with the vastus muscles via the quadriceps femoris tendon. Near its origin, the rectus femoris muscle is just deep to sartorius and tensor fasciae latae as these muscles diverge medially and laterally (respectively) from the ASIS.

Medial Compartment Muscles

Pectineus muscle originates from the pectineal line of the superior pubic ramus, just above the inguinal ligament, enters the thigh deep to the inguinal ligament, forming the medial half of the floor of the femoral triangle, and inserts on the body of the femur immediately below the lesser trochanter. The adductor longus, adductor brevis, and adductor magnus muscles originate from the pelvic bone medial to pectineus (part of the adductor magnus' origin is posterior to pectineus). Adductor longus is the most superficial of these 3 medial compartment muscles. Adductor brevis is just deep to adductor longus, and adductor magnus, in turn, is deep to adductor brevis (and its lateral-most fibers are deep to pectineus). Adductor longus originates from the superior part of the body of the pubic bone and inserts onto the middle third of the body of the femur (linea aspera) posteriorly. Adductor brevis originates from the lower part of the pubic body and adjacent ischiopubic ramus and inserts onto the proximal third of the femoral shaft (linea aspera) posteriorly. Adductor magnus originates from the ischiopubic ramus and adjacent ischial tuberosity, and inserts in 2 parts: a hamstring part and an adductor part. The hamstring part inserts onto the adductor tubercle of the medial femoral condyle and the adductor part inserts onto the body of the femur immediately lateral to the lines of insertion of adductors brevis and longus.

Nerves and Vessels

The peripheral nerves that innervate the lower limb originate from the lumbar (L1–L4) and lumbosacral plexuses (L4–S4). The main blood supply of the lower limb is provided by the femoral artery, the continuation of the external iliac artery distal to beyond the plane of the inguinal ligament. The nerves and vessels pass between the pelvis or posterior abdominal wall and the lower limb through several openings, mainly via the subinguinal space anteriorly and the greater sciatic foramen posteriorly.

Femoral Nerve

The femoral nerve, a branch of the lumbar plexus, leaves the posterior abdominal wall in a groove between iliacus and psoas major below the inguinal ligament to enter the femoral triangle. The femoral nerve innervates iliacus, pectineus (usually), sartorius, and quadriceps femoris and the cutaneous supply to areas of the anterior thigh, medial leg, and medial aspect of the foot.

Femoral Vessels

The femoral artery, the continuation of the external iliac artery as it passes under the inguinal ligament, lies just medial to the femoral nerve in the femoral triangle. The femoral vein lies just medial to the artery. Typically, in the proximal part of the femoral triangle, the femoral artery give rise to the deep femoral artery and then continues to the apex of the triangle where it enters the adductor (subsartorial) canal accompanied by the femoral vein and 2 branches of the femoral nerve, the nerve to vastus medialis and the saphenous nerve.

Lateral Femoral Cutaneous Nerve

The lateral femoral cutaneous nerve, a branch of the lumbar plexus, passes from the posterior abdominal wall to the lower limb, below the inguinal ligament, and medial to the ASIS along the superficial surface of the sartorius muscle at its origin. The nerve initially occupies a space within the fascia lata between the sartorius and tensor fasciae latae muscles and then pierces the fascia lata a few centimeters below the ASIS to supply a cutaneous area along the lateral aspect of the thigh.

Femoral Triangle

The subinguinal space is the area between the inguinal ligament (spanning between the ASIS and the pubic tubercle) and the pelvic bone, which opens from the posterior abdominal wall into a triangular depression in the proximal thigh, the femoral triangle. The inguinal ligament forms the base of the triangle, and the medial margin of sartorius muscle and the lateral margin of adductor longus muscle form its lateral and medial borders, respectively. The floor of the triangle is made up of iliacus and psoas muscles (joining to form iliopsoas) laterally and by pectineus muscle medially. The main contents of the triangle are, from lateral to medial, the femoral nerve and branches, the femoral artery and branches, the femoral vein and tributaries, and deep inguinal lymph nodes and lymphatic channels (within the femoral canal).

Technique

Anterior Superior Iliac Spine

**ANTERIOR SUPERIOR
ILIAC SPINE**
Transverse
FIG. 5.1

The patient should be supine and appropriately draped to allow for palpation of landmarks and for placing and manipulating the probe while maintaining patient privacy and comfort.

Locate the ASIS and adjacent iliac crest by palpation. Place the face of the probe transversely over the ASIS such that the probe is centered over the ASIS with the medial part of the probe face on the skin of the anterior abdominal wall and the lateral part of the probe on the skin over the anterior-most extent of the gluteal region. Identify the smooth hyperechoic arc of the ASIS and its dense acoustic shadow. On the medial side of the ASIS identify the 3 muscle layers of the anterior abdominal wall: external abdominal oblique, internal abdominal oblique, and transversus abdominis. Locate the peritoneum at the deep surface of the transversus abdominis. Observe for respiratory movements and peristalsis of abdominal contents deep to the peritoneum. On the lateral side of the ASIS identify gluteal muscles (medius and minimus) projecting anteriorly from the posterior or gluteal surface of the iliac ala. The origins of sartorius and tensor fasciae latae are difficult to identify at the ASIS, but both muscles can be readily identified by scanning a short distance (1-2 cm) inferior to the ASIS. Scan up and down along sartorius (medially and inferiorly

 Figure 5.1 Transverse view of anterior superior iliac spine (ASIS) and related muscles, including gluteus medius and minimus and abdominal wall muscles, and the origins of sartorius and tensor fasciae latae (TFL).

from the ASIS) for several centimeters. The muscle profile appears just below the ASIS, and the muscle enlarges rapidly to its familiar "strap" shape (flattened oval profile). Place the probe back over the ASIS and scan up and down over tensor fasciae latae (laterally/posteriorly and inferiorly from the ASIS) for several centimeters. Like the sartorius, the tensor fasciae latae quickly enlarges and its oval muscle tissue profile becomes obvious a very short distance below the ASIS.

Sartorius, Tensor Fasciae Latae, and Rectus Femoris

SARTORIUS TENSOR FASCIAE LATAE RECTUS FEMORIS
Transverse
FIG. 5.2

Starting with the same patient position and draping, place the probe over the ASIS and slowly slide the probe inferiorly until both tensor fasciae latae and sartorius can be identified within the image. Keeping both tensor fasciae latae and sartorius in the image, continue slowly scanning inferiorly until the rectus femoris muscle begins to appear immediately deep to these 2 muscles. After identifying the rectus femoris, slide the probe face back superiorly to the point where the rectus femoris muscle disappears and attempt to identify the hyperechoic profile and acoustic shadow of anterior inferior iliac spine. Return the probe distally to the point where tensor fasciae latae, sartorius, and rectus femoris can be clearly identified within the same image. In the medial aspect of the image, deep to sartorius and deep to the medial aspect of rectus femoris, identify the iliopsoas muscle. The hyperechoic reflection of the femoral head and proximal part of the femoral neck (viewed obliquely) covered by fibrous hip joint capsule and iliofemoral ligament can be seen just deep to iliopsoas in this position. The anterior-most extent of gluteus medius can be identified deep to tensor fasciae latae.

Lateral Femoral Cutaneous Nerve

LATERAL FEMORAL CUTANEOUS NERVE
Transverse
FIG. 5.3

Beginning with the probe in the last position above, scan slowly a short distance inferiorly until, as tensor fasciae latae moves posteriorly/laterally and sartorius moves medially, rectus femoris comes to occupy a more superficial position between these 2 muscles. Observe that the lateral femoral cutaneous nerve has pierced the deep surface of the fascia lata to occupy a small fatty compartment within the fascia lata between the tensor fasciae latae and the sartorius and just superficial to the rectus femoris. Attempt to follow the nerve until it pierces the superficial surface of the fascia lata into a cutaneous position.

Hip Joint, Iliopsoas, and Iliofemoral Ligament

HIP JOINT
Longitudinal
FIG. 5.4

The patient should be supine and appropriately draped, with the limb to be examined rotated externally. Using a curved array abdominal probe, place the probe face just below the center of the inguinal fold, oriented obliquely (roughly perpendicular to the inguinal fold) from superomedial to inferolateral. Adjust the probe position and tilt until the hyperechoic profile of the femoral head and neck can be identified. Adjust probe position and tilt until the hyperechoic profile of the acetabular rim can be seen along with the femoral head and neck. Identify the acetabular labrum projecting a short distance over the femoral head from the rim of the acetabulum. Just superficial to the acetabular rim, labrum, femoral head, and femoral neck, identify the joint capsule and iliofemoral ligament, which typically appear hypoechoic with multiple linear hyperechoic bands. The capsule and ligament begin at the acetabular margin superiorly and pass over the labrum, femoral head, and femoral neck. The capsule should be uniform in thickness (4-6 mm) and parallel to the profile of the head and neck of the femur. Superficial to the joint capsule identify the iliopsoas muscle with its characteristic hyperechoic deep tendinous part in contact with the capsule (there is an intervening iliopsoas bursa, which cannot be seen unless it is inflamed) as it passes over the hip joint and femoral neck to insert at the lesser trochanter (just out of view posteromedially in Figure 5.4). Sartorius muscle is the most superficial muscle in this view, and in the distal part of the image, a portion of rectus femoris can often be identified between sartorius and iliopsoas.

Femoral Triangle

FEMORAL TRIANGLE FEMORAL VESSELS AND NERVE
Transverse
FIG. 5.5

The patient should be supine and appropriately draped, with the limb to be examined rotated externally. Place the probe (high-frequency linear) below the inguinal fold just medial to the center of the inguinal ligament, oriented obliquely about halfway between parallel to the inguinal fold and a true horizontal plane. Adjust the probe position until the pulsating femoral artery is visible near the center of the image. Identify the iliopsoas in the floor of the triangle laterally and the pectineus in the floor of the triangle medially. Medial to the femoral artery, identify the femoral vein and observe the effects of varying probe face pressure on the vein. On the lateral side of the artery identify the femoral nerve, adjusting probe position, pressure, and tilt to

Labels on illustration:
- Fascia lata
- Tensor fasciae latae m.
- Gluteus medius m.
- Rectus femoris m.
- Iliofemoral ligament
- Sartorius m.
- Iliopsoas m.
- Head of femur

Labels on ultrasound image:
- Fascia lata
- Lateral femoral cutaneous n.
- Sartorius m.
- Tensor fasciae latae m.
- Rectus femoris m.
- Iliopsoas m.
- Gluteus medius m.
- Iliofemoral ligament
- Head of femur

Figure 5.2 Transverse view of sartorius, tensor fasciae latae, rectus femoris, and iliopsoas a short distance below anterior inferior iliac spine, crossing anterior to the femoral head.

optimize the "honeycomb" echotexture of the nerve, which commonly has a triangular profile in this view. Scan inferiorly a short distance along the femoral artery to observe its deep femoral branch. Using as little probe pressure as possible, slide the probe superiorly along the femoral vein and attempt to identify the point where the great saphenous vein enters the femoral vein through a defect in the fascia lata, the saphenous opening. Observe the motion of venous valves in the femoral vein and its tributaries.

Pectineus and Adductor Muscles in the Proximal Thigh

PECTINEUS AND ADDUCTOR MUSCLES
Transverse
FIG. 5.6

Starting from the above-mentioned probe position and orientation for viewing the contents of the femoral triangle, slide the probe medially keeping the pectineus muscle in view. Continue scanning medially until the medial edge of pectineus is just in view at the lateral aspect of the image and the 3 adductor muscles can be seen medial to pectineus. The most superficial of the 3 is the adductor longus. Immediately deep to adductor longus is adductor brevis. Deep to adductor brevis is adductor magnus. Note that the lateral-most part of adductor magnus is also deep to pectineus. Scan inferiorly and superiorly along the adductor brevis muscle and attempt to identify branches of the obturator nerve at the deep and superficial surfaces of the muscle.

Figure 5.3 Transverse view of the lateral femoral cutaneous nerve within the fascia lata between sartorius and tensor fasciae latae.

CLINICAL APPLICATIONS

US examination is commonly used in the evaluation of the painful hip resulting from musculoskeletal injuries or degenerative disorders, such as iliopsoas tendinosis/tendonitis, partial or complete tendon tears, iliopsoas bursitis, tears or cysts of the acetabular labrum, and effusions resulting from inflammatory conditions affecting the hip joint. US can also be used to guide needles for hip joint aspiration or injection of anti-inflammatory drugs and local anesthetic agents.

These techniques can be used to guide needles for access and catheter placement in the femoral vein or artery. US examination, including Doppler US, is commonly used for the detection of deep vein thrombi in lower limb veins, including the femoral vein and its tributaries. Doppler US is also used for measurement of flow velocity profiles in the femoral artery in suspected peripheral artery disease.

US-guided femoral nerve blocks are used in surgeries involving the anterior thigh and for postoperative pain control in anterior thigh and knee surgery. Femoral nerve block combined with sciatic nerve block can be used in a wide variety of lower limb surgeries. Lateral femoral cutaneous nerve blocks are used in the evaluation and management of lateral thigh pain syndromes resulting from compression or entrapment of the nerve (meralgia paresthetica).

Incidental pathologies such as femoral or inguinal hernias may also be detected during US examinations in the proximal thigh.

Sartorius m.
Iliopsoas m.
Rectus femoris m.
Rim of acetabulum
Labrum
Iliofemoral ligament
Head of femur
Neck of femur

Sartorius m.
Rectus femoris m.
Iliopsoas m.
Labrum
Iliofemoral lig.
Rim of acetabulum
Head of femur
Neck of femur

Figure 5.4 Longitudinal view of the hip joint including the rim of the acetabulum, acetabular labrum, femoral head and neck, iliofemoral ligament, and iliopsoas muscle/tendon.

Figure 5.5 Transverse view of the femoral nerve, femoral artery, and femoral vein in the femoral triangle.

Figure 5.6 Transverse view of pectineus, adductor longus, adductor brevis, and adductor magnus just medial to the femoral triangle.

Gluteal Region

Review of the Anatomy

Bones

The bones of the gluteal region are the pelvic bones, sacrum, coccyx, and greater trochanter, intertrochanteric crest, and gluteal tuberosity of the proximal femur.

Greater and Lesser Sciatic Foramina

Two ligaments, the sacrospinous and sacrotuberous, stabilize the sacrum relative to the pelvic bone and form parts of the borders of 2 openings, the greater and lesser sciatic foramina. The greater sciatic foramen is superior to the sacrospinous ligament and ischial spine, and the lesser sciatic foramen is inferior to the sacrospinous ligament and ischial spine. The bony margins of the 2 foramina are formed by the greater sciatic and lesser sciatic notches of the posterior margin of the pelvic bone. The gluteal region communicates with the pelvis through the greater sciatic foramen and with the perineum through the lesser sciatic foramen.

Muscles and Fascia

Fascia Lata and Iliotibial Tract

The fascia lata is the deep fascia of the gluteal region and thigh. The fascia lata covers only the superficial surface of gluteus medius but splits into 2 layers to cover both the deep and superficial surfaces of gluteus maximus and tensor fasciae latae. It has a thickened band laterally, the iliotibial tract, which begins proximally as fibrous extensions from the superficial and deep surfaces of gluteus maximus and from the superficial and deep surfaces of tensor fasciae latae, which join together in the anterior part of the gluteal region. The iliotibial tract continues distally along the lateral aspect of the thigh and then crosses the knee joint to attach at the anterolateral surface of the tibia.

Gluteal Maximus, Medius, and Minimus

The posterior (gluteal) surface of the ala of the ilium serves as a site of origin for gluteus maximus, medius and minimus.

Gluteus maximus is a large rhomboid-shaped muscle that originates from the posterior surface of the ilium posterior to the posterior gluteal line, the posterior surface of the sacrum, and the posterior surface of the sacrotuberous ligament and inserts into the posterior edge of the iliotibial tract and the gluteal tuberosity of the proximal femur. Gluteus maximus is the largest and most superficial muscle of the gluteal region. Gluteus medius originates from the gluteal surface of the ilium between the posterior and anterior gluteal lines and inserts onto the lateral surface of the greater trochanter of the femur. Lying deep to gluteus medius, gluteus minimus originates from the surface of the ilium between the anterior and inferior gluteal lines and inserts onto the anterior surface of the greater trochanter.

Tensor Fasciae Latae

The tensor fasciae latae originates from the iliac crest along a line between the ASIS and the tubercle of the crest and uses the iliotibial tract to gain attachment to the tibia. In this position, the tensor fasciae latae is superficial to gluteus medius and minimus.

Deep Group of Muscles

Several lateral rotators of the femur, comprising the deep group of gluteal region muscles, originate from the pelvic bone and pass through the gluteal region to insert on the proximal femur. Piriformis originates from the pelvic surface of the sacrum, enters the gluteal region through the greater sciatic foramen, and inserts onto medial surface of the apex of the greater trochanter of the femur. The obturator internus originates from the deep surface of the margin of the obturator foramen and obturator membrane, turns approximately 90 degrees over the lesser sciatic notch, and its tendon passes laterally through the floor of the gluteal region between gemellus superior and inferior muscles to insert onto the trochanteric fossa of the greater trochanter. The gemellus superior and gemellus inferior originate from the posterior surfaces of the ischial spine and tuberosity, respectively, and insert onto the intervening tendon of obturator internus and the trochanteric fossa. Quadratus femoris, the most inferior of the lateral rotators of the hip, originates from the lateral surface of the ischium adjacent to the ischial tuberosity and inserts onto the intertrochanteric crest of the femur.

Hamstring Origin

The hamstring muscles of the posterior compartment of the thigh originate from a large common tendon attached along the posterior/posterolateral surface of the ischial tuberosity.

Nerves and Arteries

Sciatic Nerve

The sciatic nerve, a major source of innervation in the lower limb, is the largest branch of the lumbosacral plexus with nerve fibers from L4 to S3. The nerve leaves the pelvis through the greater sciatic foramen inferior to piriformis and descends through the gluteal region immediately deep to the gluteus maximus and coursing over the gemellus superior, the tendon of obturator internus, inferior gemellus, and finally, the quadratus femoris. At the inferior extent of the gluteal region, the nerve is located between the gluteus maximus and the quadratus femoris, where it lies in a shallow groove between the intertrochanteric crest laterally and the ischial tuberosity medially, adjacent to the common hamstring tendon of origin. At the inferior border of quadratus femoris, the sciatic nerve enters the thigh where it continues to descend deep to the hamstring muscles of the posterior compartment of the thigh. In the distal thigh, the sciatic nerve divides into its terminal branches, the tibial and common fibular nerves.

Other Branches of the Lumbosacral Plexus

Other branches of the lumbosacral plexus that enter the gluteal region through the greater sciatic foramen include the superior gluteal nerve (gluteus medius, gluteus minimus, and tensor fasciae latae), inferior gluteal nerve (gluteus maximus), pudendal nerve (perineum), posterior femoral cutaneous nerve (cutaneous supply in the posterior thigh), the nerve to obturator internus (obturator internus and gemellus superior), and the nerve to quadratus femoris (gemellus inferior and quadratus femoris).

Superior and Inferior Gluteal Arteries

The superior and inferior gluteal arteries, branches of the internal iliac artery in the pelvis, enter the gluteal region through the greater sciatic foramen, respectively, above and below the piriformis muscle. These arteries supply muscles and other structures of the gluteal region and hip joint and provide anastomotic branches for collateral circulation with the femoral artery.

The superior gluteal artery, accompanied by the superior gluteal nerve, courses anteriorly between gluteus medius and gluteus minimus.

Technique

Anterior Gluteal Region

TENSOR FASCIA LATA
GLUTEUS
MEDIUS AND MINIMUS
Longitudinal
FIG. 5.7

For examination of the anterior gluteal region on the right, the patient should be in left lateral decubitus position and appropriately draped to allow for palpation of landmarks and probe positioning. Orient the probe in the long axis of the thigh halfway between the ASIS and the tubercle of the iliac crest, a few centimeters inferior to the crest. The probe face should be directed slightly posteriorly (as opposed to true coronal orientation). Identify the tensor fasciae latae muscle and the layers of fascia lata on its superficial and deep surfaces. Deep to the tensor fasciae latae identify the gluteus medius muscle. Deep to the gluteus medius, and with a slightly different fiber orientation and connective tissue density, identify the gluteus minimus muscle.

GLUTEUS MEDIUS
GLUTEUS MINIMUS
GLUTEAL SURFACE OF
ILIUM
Longitudinal
FIG. 5.8

From the above-mentioned position, slide the probe posteriorly, maintaining the same orientation, to just beyond the lateral/posterior border of tensor fasciae latae. Adjust the probe position slightly superiorly until, from superficial to deep, the fascia lata, gluteus medius muscle, gluteus minimus muscle, and the posterior (gluteal) surface of the iliac ala can be clearly seen and identified.

Fascia lata
Tensor fasciae latae m.
Gluteus maximus m.

Fascia lata
Tensor fasciae latae m.
Fascia lata
Gluteus medius m.
Gluteus minimus m.

Figure 5.7 Longitudinal view of tensor fasciae latae, gluteus medius, and gluteus minimus at the anterior-most extent of the gluteal region.

Greater Trochanter: Tendons of the Gluteus Medius and Minimus

ILIOTIBIAL TRACT TENDONS OF GLUTEUS MEDIUS AND MINIMUS
Transverse
FIG. 5.9

The patient should be in lateral decubitus position and appropriately draped to allow for palpation of landmarks and probe positioning. Locate the greater trochanter by palpation and place the probe transversely near its superior aspect. Identify the hyperechoic reflection and acoustic shadow of the greater trochanter and adjust the probe position as needed to obtain an image that includes the following bony features: a relatively flat lateral surface parallel to the skin (lateral surface), which ends anteriorly with a steep drop onto a surface directed anteriorly/anterolaterally (anterior surface) and which curves posteriorly onto a surface directed posterolaterally. This area of the greater trochanter is often referred to clinically as the trochanteric apex. The gluteus medius inserts onto the lateral surface, and its tendon can be seen in transverse view along the lateral surface of the trochanter. The gluteus minimus inserts onto the anterior surface, and its tendon can be seen in this position, although it is commonly hypoechoic due to **anisotropy**. The gluteus maximus crosses along the

Posterior edge of tensor fasciae latae m.

Fascia lata

Gluteus medius m.

Gluteus minimus m.

Gluteal surface of ilium

Posterior edge of tensor fasciae latae m.
Fascia lata

Gluteus medius m.

Gluteus minimus m.

Gluteal surface of ilium

 Figure 5.8 Longitudinal view of gluteus medius, gluteus minimus, and the posterior (gluteal) surface of the ala of the ilium, just posterior to the lateral/posterior border of tensor fasciae latae.

posterior surface of the greater trochanter (not a true tendinous attachment surface), separated from the bone surface by the trochanteric bursa (only visible when inflamed), and inserts into the posterior edge of the iliotibial tract of fascia lata.

TENDON OF GLUTEUS MEDIUS
Longitudinal
FIG. 5.10

Beginning from the transverse view of the greater trochanter above, center the lateral facet in the image and carefully rotate the probe 90 degrees (probe marker directed superiorly) into a longitudinal orientation over the lateral surface. Adjust the probe position as needed (usually a short distance superiorly) until the insertion of the gluteus medius tendon can be identified. Fanning and "heel-toe" tilting of the probe face are helpful to visualize the fibrillar architecture of the tendon, which may be obscured because of anisotropy. Identify the iliotibial tract overlying the tendon. Fibers of gluteus maximus muscle can also be seen inserting onto the iliotibial tract from the superior aspect of the image.

Sciatic Nerve in the Gluteal Region

SCIATIC NERVE GLUTEUS MAXIMUS QUADRATUS FEMORIS
Transverse
FIG. 5.11

The patient should be prone and appropriately draped to allow for palpation of landmarks and probe manipulation. By palpation identify the posterior edge of the greater trochanter/intertrochanteric crest laterally and the ischial tuberosity medially. Place a curved array abdominal probe, oriented transversely, between these 2 landmarks (probe marker directed laterally) and adjust the probe position until the hyperechoic profile of the intertrochanteric crest can be identified along the lateral edge

 Figure 5.9   Transverse view of the tendons of gluteus minimus and gluteus medius at the anterior and lateral surfaces of the greater trochanter. Muscle fibers of gluteus maximus are seen attaching at the posterior edge of the iliotibial tract.

of the image and the hyperechoic ischial tuberosity with the overlying hypoechoic/anechoic (due to anisotropy) common hamstring tendon can be seen at the medial aspect of the image. Identify the quadratus femoris muscle spanning between the lateral surface of the ischium adjacent to the tuberosity and the intertrochanteric crest.

Adjacent to the ischial tuberosity and common hamstring tendon, between quadratus femoris and the gluteus maximus muscle, identify the ovoid or triangular profile of the sciatic nerve with its typical hyperechoic honeycomb appearance (fanning and tilting the probe face as needed to minimize anisotropy).

CLINICAL APPLICATIONS

US examination is being increasingly used in the evaluation of lateral hip pain resulting from musculoskeletal injuries or overuse disorders, such as gluteus medius or gluteus minimus tendinosis/tendonitis, partial/complete tendon tears, or associated trochanteric bursopathy/bursitis. US is also used to guide needles for peritendinous or intrabursal injection of local anesthetics and/or anti-inflammatory steroids. Lateral "snapping" hip syndrome results from the iliotibial tract or the anterior border of gluteus maximus sliding back and forth across

the greater trochanter, and this sudden movement can be detected in real-time images as the examiner passively flexes and externally rotates the hip.

US-guided sciatic nerve blocks are used in surgeries involving the knee, posterior leg, Achilles (calcaneal) tendon, ankle, and foot and for postoperative control of posterior knee pain. Sciatic nerve block combined with femoral nerve block is used in a wide variety of lower limb surgeries.

Gluteus maximus m.

Tendon of gluteus medius

Lateral surface of greater trochanter

Gluteus maximus m.

Iliotibial tract

Tendon of gluteus medius

Lateral surface of greater trochanter

Figure 5.10 Longitudinal view of the tendon of gluteus medius inserting onto the lateral surface of the greater trochanter of the femur.

Figure 5.11 Transverse view of the sciatic nerve in the gluteal region, between gluteus maximus and quadratus femoris, and adjacent to the common hamstring tendon of origin at the ischial tuberosity.

Thigh

Review of the Anatomy

Bones

The femur is the bone of the thigh. From the junction of the femoral neck with the trochanteric region, the body of the femur descends obliquely from lateral to medial and ends at the medial and lateral condyles, which articulate with corresponding articular surfaces of the medial and lateral condyles of the tibial plateau. The proximal half of the body of the femur is triangular in profile, with smooth borders between the anterior surface and its posteromedial and posterolateral surfaces, and with a coarse ridge, the linea aspera, at its posterior border. The distal half of the body widens as it approaches the condyles, and the linea aspera divides into medial and lateral supracondylar lines, forming an additional posterior surface as the femur approaches the popliteal fossa.

Muscles and Fascia

Compartments

The muscles of the thigh are divided into 3 compartments by the fascia lata and its intermuscular septae. The anterior compartment muscles include quadriceps femoris and sartorius. The posterior compartment muscles are the hamstrings: biceps femoris, semitendinosus, and semimembranosus. The medial compartment muscles were briefly reviewed in a previous section.

Anterior Compartment

The quadriceps femoris muscle consist of rectus femoris, vastus lateralis, vastus intermedius, and vastus medialis.

- The *rectus femoris* muscle is the most superficial of the quadriceps group and the only quadriceps femoris muscle that crosses both the hip and knee joints. It originates via a straight tendon from the anterior inferior iliac spine and a second reflected tendon from the ilium just superior to the acetabulum and inserts along with the vastus muscles via the quadriceps femoris tendon onto the patella.
- *Vastus lateralis* originates from the distal inferior surface of the greater trochanter of the femur, the superolateral part of the intertrochanteric line, and from a line along the lateral lip of the linea aspera.

- *Vastus intermedius* originates from a wide area along the posterolateral surface, anterior surface, and medial border of the body of the femur, separating vastus lateralis from most of the posterolateral surface of the femur.
- *Vastus medialis* originates along a line beginning at the inferomedial aspect of the intertrochanteric line, continues along the medial lip of the linea aspera and adjacent posteromedial surface of the body of the femur, and ends in the distal femur a short distance along the medial supracondylar line. The vastus muscles, along with rectus femoris, insert onto the patella via the quadriceps femoris tendon.

Sartorius originates from the medial aspect of the ASIS and crosses the thigh from lateral to medial. In the first part of its course, sartorius forms the lateral border of the femoral triangle. Beyond the apex of the triangle, sartorius forms the roof or anterior wall of the adductor canal throughout the middle third of the thigh. Sartorius inserts on the medial surface of the proximal tibia along with gracilis and semitendinosus. The anterior compartment muscles are innervated by the femoral nerve.

The *fascia lata* is the deep fascia of the gluteal region and thigh. The fascia lata has a thickened band laterally, the *iliotibial tract*, which begins proximally in the anterior part of the gluteal region and continues distally along the vastus lateralis muscle, crosses the knee joint, and attaches to the anterolateral surface of the lateral tibial condyle.

Posterior Compartment

The 3 hamstring muscles of the posterior compartment are biceps femoris, semitendinosus, and semimembranosus.

- The long head of *biceps femoris* originates from a common tendon with semitendinosus attached to the medial half of the ischial tuberosity and inserts via a common tendon with the short head at the head of the fibula. The short head originates along a line beginning about midfemur at the lateral lip of the linea aspera and ending at the proximal part of the lateral supracondylar line. Biceps femoris is the most lateral of the posterior compartment muscles and has an oblique medial to lateral course through the thigh.

- *Semitendinosus* originates from a conjoined tendon with biceps femoris attached to the medial half of the ischial tuberosity. The muscle belly, which lies just medial to biceps femoris in the upper half of the thigh, tapers about midthigh to a long thin tendon that inserts onto the anteromedial surface of the proximal tibia along with sartorius and gracilis.
- *Semimembranosus* originates from the lateral half of the ischial tuberosity via a tendon that expands into a broad flattened aponeurosis with a prominent ovoid lateral free margin lying deep to the semitendinosus muscle belly. Muscle fibers arise from the surface of the aponeurosis and enlarge to form the belly of semimembranosus, which lies medial and deep to the semitendinosus muscle and tendon through the posterior compartment of the thigh. Just above the knee joint the muscle tapers to a thick tendon, which passes over the knee joint capsule at the medial femoral condyle and inserts onto a horizontal groove in the posteromedial aspect of the medial tibial condyle.

The posterior compartment muscles are innervated by the sciatic nerve.

Nerves and Vessels

Femoral Artery and Adductor Canal

The femoral artery is the major blood supply of the lower limb, and its course and relationships through the femoral triangle and adductor canal in the thigh are anatomically important. The femoral artery is the continuation of the external iliac artery as it passes under the inguinal ligament where it comes to lie just medial to the femoral nerve in the femoral triangle. The femoral vein lies just medial to the artery. Typically, in the proximal part of the triangle, the femoral artery gives rise to the deep femoral artery and then continues to the apex of the triangle where it enters the adductor canal.

The adductor canal begins at the apex of the femoral triangle and ends in the distal thigh at the adductor hiatus, the gap between the hamstring part of adductor magnus and the adductor part of the muscle, which opens into the popliteal fossa. The canal is roughly triangular in profile with a lateral wall formed by vastus medialis, a posteromedial wall

formed by adductor longus, and an anterior wall formed by sartorius.

The femoral artery descends in the canal accompanied by the femoral vein and 2 branches of the femoral nerve, the nerve to vastus medialis and the saphenous nerve. The femoral vessels leave the canal through the adductor hiatus, becoming the popliteal vessels. The saphenous nerve continues through the thigh along the deep surface of sartorius, emerges between sartorius and the tendon of gracilis just above the knee joint, and then pierces the deep fascia to provide cutaneous supply to the medial surface of the leg from the knee joint to the medial aspect of the foot.

The deep branch of the femoral artery descends in the thigh across pectineus, then passes posterior (deep) to the adductor longus where it first lies between adductor longus and adductor brevis, and then beyond the distal edge of adductor brevis, it lies between adductor longus and adductor magnus. In the femoral triangle, the deep femoral artery has medial and lateral femoral circumflex branches, and beyond the triangle it has 3 perforating branches, which provide arterial supply to structures of the posterior compartment.

Sciatic Nerve

The sciatic nerve continues into the thigh from the gluteal region as it passes beyond the inferior margin of quadratus femoris and comes to lie immediately anterior (deep) to biceps femoris. The nerve lies along the anteromedial surface of the long head of biceps femoris through most of the thigh and typically divides just proximal to the popliteal fossa into its terminal branches, the tibial nerve and the common fibular nerve. In the posterior compartment the sciatic nerve innervates the long head of biceps, semitendinosus, and semimembranosus via its tibial division, whereas the short head of biceps femoris receives its motor supply from the common fibular division of the nerve. The tibial nerve continues through the central part of the popliteal fossa and on into the posterior compartment of the leg. The common fibular nerve diverges laterally along the medial edge of the biceps femoris muscle and tendon, then crosses subcutaneously along the fibular neck into the lateral compartment of the leg.

Technique

Adductor Canal

FEMORAL ARTERY AND VEIN
SAPHENOUS NERVE
Transverse
FIG. 5.12

The patient should be supine with the thigh laterally rotated, appropriately draped for US examination from just below the ASIS through the proximal third of the thigh anteromedially. Place the probe in a transverse orientation just below and medial to the ASIS. Identify the sartorius and center the muscle in the image. Slide the probe distally along the oblique (lateral to medial) course of the sartorius for a short distance and observe as the muscle crosses superficially over the femoral vessels beyond the apex of the femoral triangle. Continue sliding the probe

 Figure 5.12 Transverse view of the femoral artery, femoral vein, and saphenous nerve in the adductor canal.

distally for another 2 to 4 cm until the femoral vessels can be seen to occupy a triangular cleft between sartorius anteriorly, vastus medialis laterally, and adductor longus posteromedially. Note the pulsations of the more superficial femoral artery and the effects of changing probe pressure on the femoral vein, which lies just deep to the artery. Fan and tilt the probe face (to minimize anisotropy) to identify the saphenous nerve, which usually lies immediately lateral to the artery along the deep surface of sartorius in the upper part of the canal. The deep femoral vessels may be visible in the deepest part of the image, where they are separated from the canal by the adductor longus muscle.

Quadriceps Femoris

**RECTUS FEMORIS
VASTUS MUSCLES**
Transverse
FIG. 5.13

The patient should be supine with minimal lateral rotation of the thigh. Slight flexion at the knee, supported by a small bolster behind the knee, may be help to relax the quadriceps muscles for US examination. Place the probe in a transverse orientation over the anterior surface of the midthigh and adjust probe position as necessary to center the rectus femoris muscle, the most superficial of the quadriceps group, in the image. Immediately deep to the central part of rectus femoris identify vastus intermedius and note its relationship to the anterior and posterolateral surfaces of the femur. Medial to vastus intermedius, identify vastus medialis and note its position from deep to the medial aspect of rectus femoris to the medial border and posteromedial surface of the femur. Between the lateral aspect of rectus femoris and the anterior surface of vastus intermedius identify the vastus lateralis. Most of the vastus lateralis is beyond the field of view, separated from the femur by the broad attachment of vastus intermedius to the anterior surface, lateral border, and posterolateral surface of the femur. Slide the probe distally along the rectus femoris muscle and note that rectus femoris becomes tendinous more proximally than the vastus muscles.

Iliotibial Tract

**ILIOTIBIAL TRACT
TENSOR FASCIAE
LATAE
VASTUS LATERALIS**
Longitudinal
FIG. 5.14

The patient should be supine and appropriately draped, with minimal external rotation of the thigh and the knee slightly flexed (a small bolster behind the knee may be helpful). Begin by placing the probe in a transverse orientation below the lateral aspect of the ASIS. Identify the muscle belly of the tensor fasciae latae and center the muscle in the image. Slide the probe distally a short distance while keeping the muscle centered in the image and observe that

the course of the tensor fasciae latae is slightly anterior to posterior. Carefully rotate the probe into a longitudinal orientation parallel to the muscle belly. Continue sliding the probe distally along the path of the muscle until the distal tapered end of the muscle can be clearly seen, as it inserts into the iliotibial tract. Observe that the iliotibial tract receives fibers from layers of fascia lata on both the superficial and deep surfaces of tensor fasciae latae muscle at this point. Deep to fascia lata covering the deep surface of tensor fasciae latae and then more distally, deep to the iliotibial tract, identify vastus lateralis. Deep to vastus lateralis identify the vastus intermedius, which is in contact with the surface of the body of the femur.

**ILIOTIBIAL TRACT
VASTUS LATERALIS
INTERMEDIUS**
Transverse
FIG. 5.15

The patient should be in the lateral decubitus position with the knee slightly flexed. A small bolster should be positioned between the patient's knees. Place the probe in a transverse orientation over the lateral surface of the anterior compartment at about the junction of the middle and distal thirds of the thigh. Note the multilaminar appearance (hyperechoic, hypoechoic, hyperechoic) of the iliotibial tract covering the lateral surface of vastus lateralis. The vastus intermedius can be clearly identified covering the posterolateral surface of the femur. Slide the probe a short distance posteriorly and attempt to identify the slightly rounded (teardrop) appearance of the posterior edge of the iliotibial tract as it blends with the fascia lata posteriorly.

Posterior Compartment: Hamstring Muscles and Sciatic Nerve

**HAMSTRING MUSCLES
SCIATIC NERVE**
Transverse
EFOV
FIGS. 5.16-5.19

The patient should be prone and appropriated draped to allow for palpation of landmarks and probe positioning. A small bolster placed under the distal leg/ankle may be helpful in relaxing the posterior compartment muscles. Locate the ischial tuberosity by palpation. Place the probe transversely over the tuberosity, and identify the hypoechoic hamstring tendon of origin over the hyperechoic profile of the bone (as shown in the gluteal region). Slide the probe distally a short distance until the muscle fibers of the long head of the biceps femoris and semitendinosus begin to appear, joined by a curving tendinous band. At this point, the long head of the biceps femoris should be just under cover of the inferior border of gluteus maximus muscle. Identify the sciatic nerve at the deep (anterior) surface of the biceps muscle. Slide the probe medially and identify the semitendinosus muscle covered by fascia lata posteriorly. At the deep surface of semitendinosus identify the hyperechoic aponeurotic

Vastus lateralis m.

Vastus intermedius m.

Femur

Rectus femoris m.

Vastus medialis m.

Fascia lata

Rectus femoris m.

Vastus lateralis m.

Vastus medialis m.

Vastus intermedius m.

Femur

Figure 5.13 Rectus femoris, vastus intermedius, vastus medialis, and vastus lateralis at the midthigh.

tendon of semimembranosus. Note the prominent tear-drop expansion at its lateral edge tapering to a broad flat tendon, which continues medial to the deep surface of semitendinosus, where muscle fibers of semimembranosus begin to form at the posterior surface of the tendon. The adductor magnus muscle can be seen deep to the sciatic nerve and hamstring muscles in this position. For this sequence, an extended field of view (EFOV) US image is shown to demonstrate all of these relationships in a single image, followed by 3 separate standard (non-EFOV) US

images, moving from lateral to medial, to demonstrate the same structures and their relationships.

BICEPS FEMORIS SCIATIC NERVE
Transverse
FIG. 5.20

Slide the probe laterally to center the long head of biceps femoris in the image. Next, slide the probe distally along the oblique (medial to lateral) course of the muscle. About midthigh, muscle fibers of the short head of biceps will begin to appear at the deep (anterolateral) surface of the long head.

Continue following the biceps femoris distally and observe as the muscle belly of the short head enlarges and the belly of the long head begins to taper as it approaches the common biceps insertion tendon a short distance above the popliteal fossa. The hyperechoic sciatic nerve can be seen along the deep (anteromedial) surface of the long head of biceps.

SEMIMEMBRANOSUS MUSCLE SEMITENDINOSUS TENDON
Transverse
FIG. 5.21

Return the probe to the transverse view of the hamstring muscles near their origin. Slide the probe medially to center the semitendinosus and semimembranosus muscles in the image. Next, slide the probe distally along the 2 muscles. Observe that as muscle fibers emerge from the posterior surface of the semimembranosus aponeurotic tendon, the muscle enlarges rapidly and comes to occupy a position directly deep to semitendinosus. Continuing distally, the semitendinosus muscle begins tapering to a relatively thin tendon at about the midthigh. Continue scanning distally along the semitendinosus tendon and semimembranosus muscle belly to about the junction of the middle and distal thirds of the thigh, a short distance above the popliteal fossa. Identify the fascia lata, semitendinosus tendon, and semimembranosus muscle belly.

Iliotibial tract

Tensor fasciae latae m.

Fascia lata

Fascia lata
Tensor fasciae latae m.
Iliotibial tract

Vastus lateralis m.

Vastus intermedius m.

Femur

Figure 5.14 Longitudinal view of the distal end of tensor fasciae latae and the iliotibial tract along the lateral aspect of vastus lateralis muscle in the proximal third of the thigh. Vastus intermedius is seen between the deep surface of vastus lateralis and the body of the femur.

CLINICAL APPLICATIONS

US examination is used for musculoskeletal injuries or disorders such as hamstring origin tendinosis/tendonitis, partial and complete tendon tears/avulsions, and/or muscle tears.

US examination, including Doppler US, is commonly used for detection of deep vein thrombi in lower limb veins, including the femoral vein and its tributaries. Doppler US is also used for the measurement of flow velocity profiles in the femoral artery in suspected peripheral artery disease.

US guidance is used for saphenous nerve blocks in the adductor canal. Saphenous nerve blocks are used for surgeries involving the medial leg, ankle, and foot or, more commonly, in combination with sciatic nerve block for surgeries below the knee (the saphenous nerve is the only nerve with sensory distribution below the knee that is not derived from the sciatic nerve).

Iliotibial tract
Vastus lateralis m.
Vastus intermedius m.
Femur

Iliotibial tract
Vastus lateralis m.
Vastus intermedius m.
Femur

Figure 5.15 Transverse view of the iliotibial tract along the lateral surface of vastus lateralis muscle at the junction of the middle and distal thirds of the thigh. Vastus intermedius is seen between the deep surface of vastus lateralis and the body of the femur.

Gluteus maximus m.

Semitendinosus (ST) m.

Biceps femoris m.
(long head)

Semimembranosus
and aponeurotic tendon

Sciatic n.

Conjoined tendon of
biceps femoris and ST

Adductor magnus m.

Gluteus
maximus m.

Fascia lata

Conjoined tendon of
biceps femoris & ST

ST

SM

Biceps
femoris m.

SM

Sciatic n.

Adductor
magnus m.

Figure 5.16 Transverse extended field of view (EFOV) of the hamstring muscles (long head of biceps femoris, semitendinosus, and semimembranosus) in the proximal-most part of the posterior thigh. The sciatic nerve can be seen in contact with the deep surface of biceps femoris (long head).

Gluteus maximus m.

Biceps femoris m. long head

Conjoined tendon biceps femoris & semitendinosus

Semitendinosus m.

Sciatic n.

Adductor magnus m.

Conjoined tendon biceps femoris & semitendinosus

Fascia lata

Gluteus maximus m.

Biceps femoris m. long head

Semiten-dinosus m.

Sciatic n.

Adductor magnus m.

Figure 5.17 Transverse view of the long head of biceps femoris and semitendinosus muscles joined by a curving tendinous band, in the proximal-most part of the thigh. The sciatic nerve is seen deep to the biceps femoris long head, which is partially overlapped by inferior fibers of gluteus maximus. Compare with Figure 5.16.

Figure 5.18 Transverse view of the long head of biceps femoris and semitendinosus muscles, along with the lateral ovoid edge of the aponeurotic tendon of semimembranosus, in the proximal thigh. Compare with Figure 5.16.

Fascia lata

Semimembranosus m.

Semitendinosus m.

Aponeurotic tendon of
semimembranosus

Adductor magnus m.

Figure 5.19 Transverse view of semitendinosus muscle and the aponeurotic tendon of
semimembranosus with muscle fibers forming along its posterior surface, in the
proximal thigh. Compare with Figure 5.16.

Biceps femoris m.
long head

Sciatic n.

Biceps femoris m.
short head

Vastus
intermedius m.

Femur

Fascia lata

Biceps femoris m.
long head

Biceps femoris m.
short head

Sciatic n.

Vastus
intermedius m.

Fat &
connective
tissue of
popliteal
fossa

Femur

Figure 5.20 Transverse view of the long and short heads of biceps femoris, along with the sciatic nerve, in the distal third of the thigh.

Tendon of semitendinosus

Semimembranosus m.

Fascia lata

Tendon of
semitendinosus

Semimembranosus m.

Fat & connective tissue
of popliteal fossa

Figure 5.21 Transverse view of the tendon of semitendinosus at the surface of semimembranosus muscle in the distal third of the thigh.

Knee

Review of the Anatomy

Knee Joint

The knee joint is a large complex synovial joint with articulations between the femoral condyles and corresponding surfaces of the tibial condyles and between the posterior surface of the patella and the femoral trochlea.

Bones, Articular Surfaces, and Menisci

Distally, the body of the femur widens as it approaches the medial and lateral condyles, and an additional femoral surface forms under the floor of the popliteal fossa. The femoral condyles, separated posteriorly and inferiorly by the intercondylar fossa, are joined anteriorly to form the femoral trochlea, the femoral articular surface for the **patella**. The trochlea, like the condyles, is covered by articular cartilage. The trochlea has sloping lateral and medial surfaces that form a groove along its central region and that are congruent with the medial and lateral articular facets (and intervening ridge) of the posterior surface of the patella. The condyles are rounded posteriorly and slightly flattened inferiorly where they meet articular facets of the medial and lateral condyles of the tibial plateau.

Between the tibial condyles is the intercondylar region of the tibial plateau, which has facets for attachment of the anterior and posterior horns of the medial and lateral **menisci** and for the anterior and posterior cruciate ligaments. The fibrocartilaginous menisci are semilunar in shape and wedgelike in profile with thicker outer edges and thin inner margins. They are described as having anterior and posterior horns connected by a middle portion, the body. The menisci cover large areas of the articular surfaces of the tibial condyles, intervening between the femoral and tibial condyles. The inferior surface of the lateral condyle of the tibia has an articular facet for the head of the fibula.

Below the condyles, the tibia tapers to its triangular body, with anteromedial, anterolateral, and posterior surfaces. At the proximal body anteriorly, there is an ovoid anterior prominence that tapers distally, the tibial tuberosity, which serves as the site of attachment of the patellar ligament.

Joint Capsule

The synovial membrane of the knee joint attaches above to the margins of the articular surfaces of the femoral condyles, below to the margins of the articular surfaces of the tibial condyles (and outer edges of the menisci), and anteriorly along the margins of the articular facets of the patella. It has a large superior recess, the suprapatellar bursa, which extends superiorly from between the patellar and trochlear articular surfaces to between the triangular suprapatellar fat pat and posterior surface of the quadriceps femoris tendon anteriorly and the prefemoral fat pad covering the anterior surface of the femur posteriorly.

The fibrous capsule of the knee has similar attachments as the synovial membrane with the prominent exception of its anterior femoral attachment. Anteriorly, the fibrous capsule attaches to the femoral body several centimeters above the articular margin of the trochlea, accommodating the suprapatellar bursa of synovial membrane. The fibrous membrane is incompletely lined by synovial membrane, separated from the synovial membrane in several sites by fat pads, including the suprapatellar fat pad at the superior pole of the patella and the infrapatellar fat pad (of Hoffa), which intervenes between the 2 membranes anteriorly, behind the patellar ligament. The fibrous capsule is reinforced by fibrous extensions from vastus medialis and lateralis, the quadriceps femoris tendon, the semimembranosus tendon, the tibial collateral ligament, and the iliotibial tract.

Ligaments

Tibial Collateral Ligament

The tibial collateral ligament of the knee is a long (8-10 cm) flattened band attached superiorly to the medial epicondyle of the femur. The ligament passes across the medial surface of the knee joint and attaches distally to the anteromedial surface of the body of the tibia 4 to 5 cm below the tibiofemoral joint line. The ligament is described as having superficial and deep layers. The superficial layer (tibiofemoral ligament), often referred to as the vertical component of the tibial collateral ligament, is the main structural component of the ligament. It is fused with the overlying deep fascia. The deep layer is fused with the underlying fibrous capsule of the knee joint, which also attaches along the outer margin of the body of medial meniscus, resulting in attachment of the tibial collateral ligament to the body of the medial meniscus. There are short extensions superiorly and inferiorly from the deep layer, the meniscofemoral and meniscotibial ligaments. Just below the tibial condyle, the ligament crosses over the medial inferior genicular vessels. Near its inferior end, the ligament is partly overlapped by the attachments of the tendons of sartorius, gracilis, and semitendinosus (pes anserinus). The tibial collateral ligament resists valgus stress at the knee joint.

Fibular Collateral Ligament

The fibular collateral ligament of the knee is a narrow, rounded cord that attaches superiorly to the lateral epicondyle of the femur just above the groove for the popliteus tendon, crosses the lateral aspect of the knee joint directed slightly posteriorly and attaches below to the lateral surface of the fibular head, along with the biceps femoris tendon. The fibular collateral ligament is separated from the fibrous capsule of the knee joint by a bursa (i.e., is not attached to the capsule or lateral meniscus). The fibular collateral ligament resists varus stress at the knee joint.

Tendons

Multiple muscles cross and act on the knee joint including the quadriceps femoris anteriorly and the hamstrings and gastrocnemius muscles posteriorly. The iliotibial tract also crosses the knee joint at its lateral aspect.

Quadriceps Femoris

The quadriceps femoris tendon is a thick strong tendon formed by contributions from rectus femoris and the vastus muscles. The tendon is commonly described as trilaminar with a superficial layer formed by rectus femoris, an intermediate layer formed by vastus lateralis and medialis, and a deep layer formed by vastus intermedius. The quadriceps femoris tendon attaches to the superior surface of the patella, which is in turn attached to the tibial tuberosity via the patellar ligament.

Iliotibial Tract

The iliotibial tract courses distally along the vastus lateralis muscle, crosses the tibiofemoral joint laterally, and attaches to Gerdy's tubercle at the anterolateral surface of the lateral tibial condyle. The posterior edge of the iliotibial tract near its tibial attachment lies a short distance anterior to the fibular collateral ligament.

Hamstring Tendons

Biceps Femoris

From the posterior compartment of the thigh, the long and short heads of biceps femoris converge distally to insert onto the lateral surface of the fibular head via a round cordlike common tendon. The tendon is readily palpable at the posterolateral aspect of the knee for several centimeters proximal to the head of the fibula.

Semimembranosus

Medially, just above the knee joint, the semimembranosus muscle tapers to a thick tendon that passes over the knee joint capsule at the medial femoral condyle alongside the medial head of gastrocnemius and inserts mainly onto a groove in the posteromedial aspect of the medial tibial condyle and partly into the fibrous joint capsule of the knee via fibrous expansions.

Semitendinosus

Semitendinosus muscle tapers to a long thin tendon just beyond midthigh. The semitendinosus tendon continues distally along the superficial surface of semimembranosus and crosses the knee joint posteromedially accompanying the tendons of gracilis and sartorius to insert on the anteromedial surface of the body of the tibia near the inferior end of the tibial collateral ligament.

Posterior Compartment of the Leg

The posterior compartment of the leg has superficial and deep muscle groups. Because of its relationship to the knee joint, an overview of the superficial muscle group (plus popliteus muscle and tendon) is provided here. The superficial muscles of the posterior leg include the medial and lateral heads of gastrocnemius, soleus, and plantaris.

Gastrocnemius

The 2 heads of the gastrocnemius along with soleus form the triceps surae muscle, which inserts onto calcaneus via the thick strong calcaneal (Achilles) tendon. The medial head of the gastrocnemius originates from the posterior surface of the femur just above the medial condyle. The thick tendinous medial edge of the muscle lies alongside the tendon of the semimembranosus just outside the joint capsule over the medial condyle. The lateral head of the gastrocnemius originates from the posterior surface of the femur just above the lateral condyle. The small plantaris muscle originates from the lateral supracondylar line just above the origin of the lateral head of gastrocnemius. The 2 heads of the gastrocnemius converge at the inferior extent of the popliteal fossa forming the belly (gaster) of the calf contour and then taper to a broad flattened tendinous band about midleg.

Soleus

Soleus muscle, deep to the gastrocnemius, originates from the posterior surfaces of the fibula and tibia and an intervening tendinous arch. In the distal leg the tendon of soleus fuses with the overlying tendon of gastrocnemius to form the calcaneal tendon. Part of the small muscle belly of the plantaris and its long thin tendon pass between the gastrocnemius and soleus to insert along the medial aspect of the calcaneal tendon.

Popliteus

In the deep group of muscles, which includes popliteus, tibialis posterior, flexor digitorum longus, and flexor hallucis longus, popliteus is particularly relevant to a discussion of the knee. The popliteus tendon attaches to the anterior part of the groove for popliteus on the lateral surface of the lateral femoral epicondyle, just below the proximal attachment of the fibular collateral ligament. Within the groove, the tendon is inside the fibrous capsule of the knee and surrounded by a small recess of the synovial space (popliteal recess). The tendon crosses the knee joint across the posterolateral aspect of the lateral meniscus and emerges from the fibrous capsule at its inferior attachment. The tendon then expands into the fan-shaped belly of popliteus, which attaches to the posterior surface of the body of the tibia above the soleal line.

Popliteal Fossa and Contents

Popliteal Fossa

The popliteal fossa is a diamond-shaped space posterior to the knee joint, formed by the muscles of the posterior compartments of the thigh and leg, through which major neurovascular structures cross between the thigh and the leg. The upper borders of the fossa are formed by biceps femoris laterally and semimembranosus and semitendinosus medially. The lower borders are formed by the medial and lateral heads of gastrocnemius muscle. The floor of the fossa is formed by the capsule of the knee joint and posterior surface of the femur, and the roof is formed by skin, superficial fascia, and popliteus muscle.

Popliteal Vessels

The femoral artery becomes the popliteal artery as it leaves the subsartorial canal and enters the popliteal fossa through the adductor hiatus of adductor magnus. The popliteal vein lies superficial to the artery in the fossa and becomes the femoral vein when it leaves the fossa through the adductor hiatus to enter the subsartorial canal.

Sciatic Nerve

The sciatic nerve approaches the popliteal fossa along the deep surface of biceps femoris. Typically, the sciatic nerve divides into its terminal branches, the tibial and common fibular nerves, just proximal to the popliteal fossa. The tibial nerve travels through the central part of the fossa, immediately superficial to the popliteal vein, whereas the common fibular nerve diverges laterally along the medial margin of biceps femoris and its tendon.

Tibial Nerve

The tibial nerve and popliteal vessels pass between the medial and lateral heads of gastrocnemius and under the tendinous arch of soleus to enter the posterior compartment of the leg at the inferior extent of the popliteal fossa, passing superficial to popliteus muscle and deep to triceps surae. The popliteal artery has genicular branches in its course through the fossa and divides into its terminal branches, the anterior and posterior tibial arteries, shortly after entering the posterior compartment of the leg.

Common Fibular Nerve

The common fibular nerve follows the biceps tendon to the posterolateral aspect of the fibular head. The nerve then crosses the neck of the fibula subcutaneously and divides into its terminal divisions, the deep and superficial fibular nerves, which enter the anterior and lateral compartments of the leg, respectively.

Technique

Suprapatellar Knee

QUADRICEPS FEMORIS TENDON SUPERIOR POLE OF PATELLA
Longitudinal
FIG. 5.22

The patient should be supine with minimal thigh rotation, and the knee should be flexed over a small bolster placed behind the knee. Place the probe in a longitudinal orientation over the distal end of the quadriceps femoris tendon in the midline of the thigh just above the patella. Identify the hyperechoic fibrillar appearance of the quadriceps femoris tendon and slide the probe distally until the attachment of the tendon to the superior pole of the patella can be seen. The patella can be readily identified by its hyperechoic bony surface and dense acoustic shadow. At the superior pole of the patella, immediately deep to the quadriceps femoris tendon, identify the generally hyperechoic triangular profile of the suprapatellar fat pad. Along the anterior surface of the femur, identify the hyperechoic prefemoral fat pad. Concentrating on the space between the 2 fat pads, slide the probe face medially and laterally until the anechoic/hypoechoic synovial fluid within the suprapatellar bursa can be clearly identified.

FEMORAL TROCHLEA QUADRICEPS FEMORIS TENDON
Transverse
FIG. 5.23

Ask the patient to flex the knee as much as comfortably possible, placing the sole of the foot on the examination table. Place the probe transversely over the anterior surface of the knee, just proximal to the patella. Identify the sloping medial and lateral bony surfaces of the femoral trochlea covered by an anechoic layer of hyaline cartilage. The lateral surface of the trochlea tends to be longer and steeper than the medial surface. Superficial to the articular cartilage identify the large hyperechoic quadriceps femoris tendon. Fanning/tilting the probe face will alter the

Tendon of quadriceps — Patella
Suprapatellar fat pad
Prefemoral fat pad
Suprapatellar bursa
Diaphysis of femur

Crural fascia
Tendon of quadriceps
Patella
Suprapatellar fat pad
Prefemoral fat pad
Suprapatellar bursa
Diaphysis of femur

Figure 5.22 Longitudinal view of the quadriceps femoris tendon, superior pole of the patella, suprapatellar fat pad, suprapatellar bursa, and prefemoral fat pad.

echogenicity of the tendon from anechoic to hyperechoic (because of anisotropy). At the medial side of the tendon, look for distal muscle tissue of vastus medialis joining the tendon.

Infrapatellar Knee

INFERIOR POLE OF PATELLA
PATELLAR LIGAMENT
Longitudinal
FIG. 5.24

The patient should be supine with the knee flexed over a small bolster placed under the knee and with minimal thigh rotation. Place the probe longitudinally over the patellar ligament at the inferior pole of the patella. Adjust the probe position until the inferior pole of the patella and the attaching fibers of the patellar ligament are clearly seen at the superior aspect of the image. Identify the hyperechoic fibrillar appearance of the ligament spanning across the image (the tibia and distal attachment of the tendon are just beyond the inferior extent of the image). Deep to the patellar tendon and fibrous joint capsule is the large infrapatellar fat pad (of Hoffa) with its hypoechoic fat mixed with hyperechoic strands of connective tissue fibers. Distal to the acoustic shadow of the patella, in the deep central part of the image, the hyperechoic bony profile of the femoral trochlea covered by anechoic hyaline cartilage can be seen.

PATELLAR LIGAMENT
TIBIAL TUBEROSITY
Longitudinal
FIG. 5.25

Next, slide the probe distally along the patellar ligament until the hyperechoic anterior surface of the tibia leading inferiorly to the rounded prominence of the tibial tuberosity with attaching fibers of the ligament can be clearly seen and identified. The deep infrapatellar bursa is located between the posterior surface of the tendon and the tibia just proximal to the tuberosity. The bursa is often difficult to identify when it is not inflamed. Deep to the patellar ligament and fibrous joint capsule, the inferior extent of the infrapatellar fat pad is readily identifiable.

Collateral Ligaments and Iliotibial Tract

TIBIAL COLLATERAL LIGAMENT
Longitudinal
FIG. 5.26

The patient should be supine with the thigh externally rotated and the knee flexed over a small bolster. Place the probe longitudinally over the medial knee, centered across the tibiofemoral joint line. Adjust the probe position and tilt until the hyperechoic profile of the medial femoral condyle proximally and the medial tibial condyle distally can be seen and identified. In the joint space between the femur and tibia, identify the wedge-shaped slightly hyperechoic

Crural fascia

Tendon of quadriceps femoris

Articular cartilage

Trochlea of femur

Crural fascia
Tendon of quadriceps femoris
Vastus medialis m.
Trochlea of femur
Articular cartilage
Trochlea of femur

Figure 5.23 Transverse view of the articular surface of the femoral trochlea, the quadriceps femoris tendon, and distal muscle fibers of vastus medialis.

profile of the body of the medial meniscus (tilting and fanning the probe face as needed to minimize anisotropy). In contact with the superficial surface of the meniscus, locate the hyperechoic deep layer of the tibial collateral ligament and its superior and inferior extensions, the meniscofemoral and meniscotibial ligaments. Superficial to the deep layer, identify the slightly less echogenic fibrillar pattern of the superficial layer of the ligament spanning across the entire image. The attachments of the superficial layer are beyond the superior and inferior edges of the image. A small bursa can sometimes be seen between the superficial and deep layers of the ligament. The superficial layer is covered by, and fused with, hyperechoic deep fascia. Sliding the probe distally while concentrating on the superficial layer of the tibial collateral ligament, attempt to follow the ligament to its attachment at the anteromedial surface of the tibia several centimeters below the joint line.

slightly flexed. By palpation, locate the biceps femoris tendon posteriorly just proximal to the fibular head. Slide fingers anteriorly from the tendon across a soft depression leading to a firm edge, the posterior edge of the iliotibial tract. Place the probe longitudinally just anterior to and parallel with the edge of the iliotibial tract. Identify the characteristic laminar appearance (hyperechoic superficial surface, hypoechoic central part, hyperechoic deep surface) of the distal iliotibial tract. Continue sliding distally toward the anterolateral surface of the lateral tibial condyle until the rounded prominence of Gerdy's tubercle can be seen. Observe that the central hypoechoic part of the iliotibial tract expands over the surface of the tubercle where it attaches. In the proximal part of the image, deep to the iliotibial tract, the tibiofemoral joint, body/anterior horn of the lateral meniscus and inferior lateral genicular vessels can be seen.

ILIOTIBIAL TRACT ATTACHMENT Longitudinal **FIG. 5.27**	The patient should be in the lateral decubitus position with a pillow or small bolster between the knees. The hip and knee joints should be

FIBULAR COLLATERAL LIGAMENT TENDON OF POPLITEUS Longitudinal **FIG. 5.28**	By palpation, locate the head of the fibula, the tendon of biceps femoris, and the posterior edge of the iliotibial tract. Place the probe longitudinally over the

 Figure 5.24 Longitudinal view of the inferior pole of the patella, patellar ligament, infrapatellar fat pad (of Hoffa), and femoral trochlea.

Figure 5.25 Longitudinal view of the patellar ligament and its insertion at the tibial tuberosity.

lateral surface of the lateral femoral condyle just posterior to the edge of the iliotibial tract with the probe marker directed superiorly and the heel of the probe face directed toward the head of the fibula. Maintaining the same orientation, adjust the probe position until the groove for popliteus along the lateral surface of the lateral femoral condyle can be clearly identified. This bony landmark is critical for locating the proximal attachment of the small cordlike fibular collateral ligament. Fanning and tilting the probe face in this position, locate the hyperechoic popliteus tendon within the groove. Immediately superior to the groove, the hyperechoic fibers of the fibular collateral ligament can be seen attaching to the surface of the lateral epicondyle and then narrowing into the cordlike central part of the ligament over the groove for popliteus. The ligament is separated from the popliteus tendon by the fibrous joint capsule. Attempt to follow the ligament distally to the fibular head. Take care not to misidentify the iliotibial tract (just anterior to the ligament) or the biceps femoris tendon (just posterior to the ligament) as the fibular collateral ligament. At the lateral surface of the head of the fibula the fibular collateral ligament fibers merge with fibers of the biceps femoris tendon.

Popliteal Fossa

TIBIAL NERVE
COMMON FIBULAR
NERVE
POPLITEAL VESSELS
Transverse
FIG. 5.29

The patient should be prone with a small bolster placed under the distal leg to slightly flex the knee, relaxing the posterior muscles around the knee joint. Place the probe transversely over the biceps femoris muscle superior to the popliteal fossa. Identify the hyperechoic honeycomb appearance of the sciatic nerve deep to muscle, along its anteromedial surface. Adjust the probe position to center the nerve in the image. Concentrating on the nerve, slide the probe distally toward the popliteal fossa until the nerve can be seen to divide into a smaller lateral branch, the common fibular nerve, and a larger medial branch, the tibial nerve. Typically, this division occurs just proximal to the popliteal fossa. Continuing to slide a short distance distally, observe that the tibial nerve descends more or less vertically into the fossa, whereas the common fibular nerve moves laterally to a position along the medial edge of biceps femoris muscle. Keeping the tibial nerve near the center of the image, apply as little pressure as possible to the probe face to avoid compression/effacement of the popliteal vein, which lies immediately deep to the tibial nerve.

Superficial layer of TCL
Deep layer of TCL
Crural fascia
Medial meniscofemoral (MF) ligament
Medial meniscus
Meniscotibial (MT) ligament
Medial condyle of femur
Medial condyle of tibia

Crural fascia
Superficial layer of TCL
Deep layer of TCL
MF lig.
MT lig.
Medial condyle of femur
Medial condyle of tibia
Medial meniscus

 Figure 5.26 Longitudinal view of the tibial collateral ligament of the knee and the body of the medial meniscus.

Iliotibial (IT) tract
Inferior lateral genicular a.
Lateral condyle of femur
Lateral meniscus
Gerdy's tubercle of lateral condyle of tibia

Inferior lateral genicular a.
IT tract
Lateral condyle of femur
Lateral meniscus
Gerdy's tubercle of lateral condyle of tibia

Figure 5.27 Longitudinal view of the iliotibial tract crossing the knee joint to its attachment at the anterolateral surface of the lateral tibial condyle (Gerdy's tubercle).

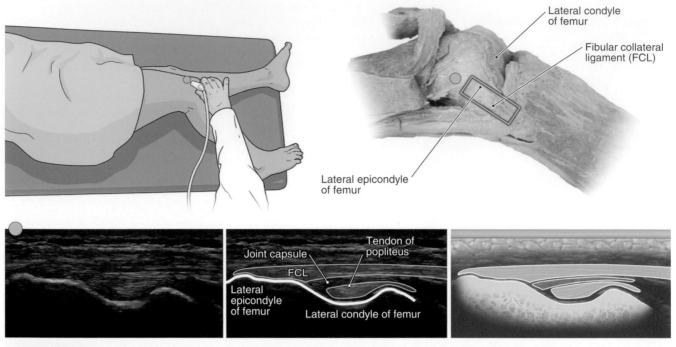

Figure 5.28 Longitudinal view of the femoral attachment of the fibular collateral ligament and the tendon of popliteus.

Figure 5.29 Transverse view of the sciatic nerve dividing into the tibial and common fibular nerves, popliteal vein, and popliteal artery in the superior part of the popliteal fossa.

Passively flexing the knee to 90 degrees may also help to fill the vein by increasing venous return from the foot and leg. Gently squeezing the calf muscles will also briefly fill the vein. Deep to the vein, look for pulsations of the popliteal artery.

POPLITEAL ARTERY POPLITEUS MUSCLE
Longitudinal
FIG. 5.30

Center the popliteal artery in the image and carefully rotate the probe into a longitudinal orientation over the artery. Slide the probe distally along the artery through and just beyond the popliteal fossa. Locate the hyperechoic bony profile of the tibial plateau sloping down to the posterior surface of the proximal body of the tibia, which is covered by the popliteus muscle belly. The popliteal artery can be seen coursing over the popliteus muscle and deep to the lateral head of gastrocnemius and then soleus as it enters the posterior compartment of the leg.

SEMIMEMBRANOSUS TENDON MEDIAL FEMORAL CONDYLE
Transverse
FIG. 5.31

Place the probe transversely over the medial aspect of the thigh above the popliteal fossa. Identify the oval profile of the semimembranosus muscle with the tendon of semitendinosus at

Crural fascia
Gastrocnemius m.
Soleus m.
Popliteal a.
Tibial plateau
Popliteus m.
Posterior surface of tiba

Crural fascia
Gastrocnemius m.
Popliteal a.
Soleus m.
Tibial plateau
Popliteus m.
Posterior surface of tiba

 Figure 5.30 Longitudinal view of the popliteal artery as it exits the popliteal fossa to enter the posterior compartment of the leg.

its posterior surface and center them in the image. Slide the probe distally along the muscle and tendon until semimembranosus can be seen to taper to a broad thick tendon. Continuing distally a short distance, observe that the semimembranosus tendon crosses behind the medial condyle in contact with the fibrous joint capsule. Immediately lateral to the tendon in this position, identify the hypoechoic medial tendinous edge and muscle tissue of medial gastrocnemius. The semimembranosus

tendon is separated from the tendinous edge of medial gastrocnemius by a (normally) thin bursa communicating with the knee joint. The tendon of semitendinosus can be seen superficial to the semimembranosus tendon. At the medial aspect of the image (adjust probe position as needed) the small gracilis tendon can be found at the posterolateral edge of sartorius. Sartorius is still muscular at this point but quickly tapers to a thin tendon distally.

 Figure 5.31 Transverse view of the tendon of semimembranosus adjacent to the medial tendinous edge of the medial head of gastrocnemius, posterior to the medial femoral condyle.

CLINICAL APPLICATIONS

US examination is used in the evaluation of several potential causes of a painful knee, mainly related to the external structures of the knee joint. These techniques are useful for evaluating disorders including tendonitis/tendinosis and partial or complete muscle/tendon tears (quadriceps femoris, patellar ligament, semitendinosus, semimembranosus, gracilis, and biceps femoris), bursitis/bursopathy (prepatellar bursa, deep infrapatellar bursa, semimembranosus-gastrocnemius bursa, and Baker's cyst), and ligamentous injuries (tibial collateral ligament, fibular collateral ligament, and iliotibial tract). US is useful for evaluating and detecting even very small knee joint effusions and for needle guidance into the suprapatellar bursa (this bursa is continuous with the knee joint proper so is not a true bursa) of the knee joint to aspirate fluid and/or to inject anti-inflammatory steroids and local anesthetic agents. Evaluation of the hyaline cartilage of the femoral trochlea can be used to detect cartilage thinning, marginal erosions, and/or increased echogenicity as a marker for the extent of cartilage loss/changes in the knee as a result of osteoarthritis or other inflammatory arthropathies. Because of acoustic shadowing behind bony surfaces, US has more limited usefulness for the evaluation of the cruciate ligaments and the menisci, although tears involving the meniscal bodies and meniscal cysts are often visible.

US examination, including Doppler US, is commonly used for the detection of deep vein thrombi in lower limb veins, including the popliteal vein and its tributaries. Doppler US is also used for the measurement of flow velocity profiles in the popliteal artery in suspected peripheral artery disease and for the detection and measurement of popliteal artery aneurysms.

US-guided sciatic nerve blocks are used in surgeries involving the knee, posterior leg, Achilles (calcaneal) tendon, ankle, and foot and for postoperative control of posterior knee pain.

Leg

Review of the Anatomy

Bones

The bones of the leg are the tibia and fibula.

Tibia

The tibia, which forms the distal part of the knee joint and most of the proximal part of the ankle joint, is the large weight-bearing bone of the leg. The body of the tibia is triangular in profile, with the posterior, anterolateral, and anteromedial surfaces delineated by anterior, medial, and interosseous (lateral) borders. The anteromedial surface is subcutaneous throughout its length. The expanded distal end of the tibia forms the superior and medial (medial malleolus) surfaces of the bony arch of the ankle joint, articulating with the upper surface (trochlea) of the talus.

Fibula

The non-weight-bearing fibula is a much smaller bone. At its proximal end, the head of the fibula articulates with a facet on the inferior surface of the lateral tibial condyle. The neck of the fibula is continuous with the body, which is triangular in profile with the posterior, lateral, and medial surfaces delineated by anterior, lateral, and medial borders. Along the medial surface is an additional border, the interosseous crest, representing the line of attachment of the tibiofibular interosseous membrane, which spans between the fibula and the interosseous border of the tibia. The fibula expands distally to the lateral malleolus, which forms the lateral surface of the ankle joint.

Muscles

The deep (crural) fascia and its intermuscular septae, along with the tibiofibular interosseous membrane, divide the leg into 3 muscular compartments: anterior, posterior, and lateral.

Anterior Compartment

The anterior compartment muscles, innervated by the deep fibular nerve, are tibialis anterior, extensor digitorum longus, fibularis tertius, and extensor hallucis longus.

Tibialis Anterior

Tibialis anterior originates from the upper two-thirds of the lateral surface of the body of the fibula, the adjacent interosseous membrane, and the surrounding deep fascia. It becomes tendinous in the distal third of the leg, crosses the ankle joint deep to the extensor retinacula, and turns under the medial side of the foot to insert at the base of the first metatarsal and adjacent plantar surface of medial cuneiform. Tibialis anterior extends (dorsiflexes) and inverts the foot.

Extensor Digitorum Longus

Extensor digitorum longus originates from the lateral tibial condyle, the medial surface of the fibular shaft and adjacent upper part of the interosseous membrane, the anterior intermuscular septum, and the surrounding deep fascia. Its tendon forms in the distal leg and crosses the ankle joint deep to the extensor retinacula. On the dorsum of the foot, the tendon divides into 4 slips that insert into the extensor expansions of the lateral toes. Extensor digitorum longus dorsiflexes the foot and extends at the joints of the lateral toes.

Fibularis Tertius

Fibularis tertius originates from the medial surface of the fibula just below extensor digitorum longus, and the 2 muscles are usually joined. On the dorsum of the foot, the tendon of fibularis tertius separates from the digital extensor tendon and inserts over the dorsal surface of the base of the fifth metatarsal distal to the insertion of fibularis brevis. This small muscle assists in dorsiflexion and eversion of the foot. This muscle is often absent.

Extensor Hallucis Longus

Extensor hallucis longus originates from the middle third of the medial surface of the fibula and adjacent interosseous membrane, between the origins of tibialis anterior medially and extensor digitorum longus laterally. At its origin, extensor hallucis longus is covered by these 2 muscles, emerging between the 2 in the distal leg to cross the ankle joint between their tendons.

Lateral Compartment

The 2 lateral compartment muscles, fibularis longus and brevis, are innervated by the superficial fibular nerve. They evert the foot and assist in plantarflexion at the ankle joint. Fibularis longus additionally assists, along with tibialis anterior and posterior, in dynamic support of the transverse arch of the foot.

Fibularis Longus

Fibularis longus, which is superficial to fibularis brevis, originates from the lateral surface of the head of the fibula, the upper half of the lateral surface of the body of the fibula, the anterior and posterior intermuscular septae that bound the compartment, and from the surrounding deep fascia. Fibularis longus becomes tendinous about midleg, and the long tendon descends along the superficial surface of the fibularis brevis muscle. In the distal third of the leg, the fibularis longus tendon descends along the posterior surface of the fibula and lateral malleolus where it is immediately posterolateral to the tendon of fibularis brevis as both tendons cross the ankle joint.

Fibularis Brevis

Fibularis brevis originates from the distal two-thirds of the lateral surface of the body of the fibula, the anterior and posterior intermuscular septae, and from the surrounding deep fascia. The muscle becomes tendinous as it descends along the posterior surface of the distal fibula and lateral malleolus, as it crosses the ankle joint with the tendon of fibularis longus.

Posterior Compartment

The posterior compartment muscles, innervated by the tibial nerve, are arranged in superficial and deep layers.

Superficial Layer

The muscles of the superficial group include the medial and lateral heads of gastrocnemius, soleus, and plantaris, all of which insert via the calcaneal tendon onto the posterior surface of calcaneus to plantarflex the foot. The 2 heads of gastrocnemius plus the small plantaris muscle cross the knee joint from their origins and therefore flex the leg.

Gastrocnemius
The medial head of gastrocnemius originates from the posterior surface of the femur just above the medial condyle, and the lateral head originates from the posterior surface of the femur just above the lateral condyle. The plantaris muscle originates from the lateral supracondylar line just above the lateral head of gastrocnemius. The 2 heads of gastrocnemius converge at the inferior extent of the popliteal fossa and then taper to a broad flattened tendinous band (gastrocnemius aponeurosis) at about midleg.

Soleus
Soleus muscle, deep to gastrocnemius, originates from the posterior surface of the head, neck, and proximal third of the fibula, from the soleal line of the posterior surface of the tibia, and from an intervening tendinous arch. The tendon of soleus fuses with the overlying tendon of gastrocnemius to complete the formation of the calcaneal tendon in the distal third of the leg.

Plantaris
The long thin plantaris tendon courses between gastrocnemius and soleus to insert along the posteromedial aspect of the calcaneal tendon.

Deep Layer

The muscles of the deep group include popliteus, tibialis posterior, flexor digitorum longus, and flexor hallucis longus. The popliteus muscle is a short muscle related to the knee joint and was previously discussed along with structures of the knee. The tendons tibialis posterior, flexor digitorum longus, and flexor hallucis longus cross the medial side of the ankle joint through the tarsal tunnel to enter the plantar aspect of the foot. The detailed anatomy of the tarsal tunnel and its contents is discussed along with structures of the ankle.

Tibialis posterior originates from the upper half of the interosseous membrane and adjacent surfaces of the tibia and fibula, between the origins of flexor hallucis longus laterally and flexor digitorum longus medially. Flexor hallucis longus originates from the middle half of the posterior surface of the body of the fibula and adjacent interosseous membrane. Flexor digitorum longus originates from the middle third of the posterior surface and lateral border of the tibia. All 3 tendons cross the ankle joint into the plantar aspect of the foot through the tarsal tunnel on the medial side of the ankle.

Kager's Fat Pad

Kager's fat pad is located in the distal leg and posterior to the ankle joint. The fat pad has a triangular shape, with the base formed by the superior cortical surface of calcaneus, the anterior border formed by flexor hallucis longus muscle and tendon, and the posterior border formed by the anterior surface of the calcaneal tendon. The apex of the triangle extends superiorly between the distal fibers of soleus and the muscles of the deep group.

Vessels and Nerves

The major neurovascular structures of the leg enter the leg from the thigh by passing through the popliteal fossa.

Popliteal Vessels

The femoral artery becomes the popliteal artery as it leaves the adductor canal of the thigh and enters the popliteal fossa through the adductor hiatus. The accompanying popliteal vein becomes the femoral vein when it leaves the fossa through the adductor hiatus to enter the adductor canal. The popliteal artery, along with the vein and tibial nerve, descends through the popliteal fossa and enters the posterior compartment of the leg by passing deep to gastrocnemius and the tendinous arch of soleus. The artery ends just beyond the tendinous arch of soleus by dividing into its terminal branches, the anterior and posterior tibial arteries.

Anterior Tibial Artery

The anterior tibial artery leaves the posterior compartment to enter the anterior compartment by passing over the superior edge of the tibiofibular interosseous membrane. The anterior tibial artery continues through the anterior compartment and ends by changing its name to the dorsalis pedis artery after crossing the ankle joint onto the dorsum of the foot.

Posterior Tibial Artery

Near its origin the posterior tibial artery has an important lateral branch, the fibular artery, which descends in the lateral aspect of posterior compartment giving perforating branches to supply the tissues of the lateral compartment, through which no artery runs. The posterior tibial artery continues through the posterior compartment along with the tibial nerve between the superficial and deep muscle layers and then leaves the leg through the tarsal tunnel to enter the foot.

Sciatic Nerve

The sciatic nerve approaches the popliteal fossa from the deep surface of biceps femoris and divides into its terminal branches, the tibial and common fibular nerves, just proximal to the popliteal fossa.

Tibial Nerve

The tibial nerve travels through the central part of the fossa between the medial and lateral heads of gastrocnemius muscle and enters the posterior compartment of the leg by passing under the tendinous arch of the soleus muscle, accompanied by the popliteal vessels. The tibial nerve descends through the posterior compartment of the leg between the superficial and deep layers of muscles, providing motor innervation to the muscles of the posterior compartment of the leg. Along with the posterior tibial vessels, the tibial nerve leaves the leg to enter the foot through the tarsal tunnel.

Sural Nerve

The medial sural cutaneous nerve branches from the tibial nerve in the popliteal fossa and, along with a communicating branch from the lateral sural cutaneous nerve (from the common fibular nerve), forms the sural nerve. The sural nerve joins the small saphenous vein in the shallow groove between the medial and lateral heads of gastrocnemius and pierces the crural fascia at about midleg to provide cutaneous innervation to the distal half of the posterolateral leg and lateral side of the foot.

Common Fibular Nerve

In the proximal part of the popliteal fossa, the common fibular branch of the sciatic diverges laterally along the medial margin of biceps femoris and its tendon, following the tendon to the posterolateral aspect of the fibular head. The nerve then crosses the fibular neck subcutaneously and enters the lateral compartment between attachments of fibularis longus muscle and divides into its terminal divisions, the deep and superficial fibular nerves.

Superficial Fibular Nerve

The superficial fibular nerve descends in the lateral compartment (supplying motor innervation to the compartment) deep to fibularis longus and then emerges between fibularis brevis and extensor digitorum longus in the distal third of the leg where it pierces the deep fascia to provide cutaneous innervation to the anterolateral surface of the leg distally and to most of the dorsum of the foot.

Deep Fibular Nerve

The deep fibular nerve pierces the anterior intermuscular septum to enter the anterior compartment where it accompanies the anterior tibial vessels. The deep fibular nerve supplies the muscles of the anterior compartment, crosses the ankle joint onto the dorsum of the foot accompanying dorsalis pedis artery, supplies motor branches to extensor digitorum brevis and extensor hallucis brevis, and then pierces the deep fascia between the first and second metatarsal bones to supply cutaneous innervation to the web space between the great and second toes.

Technique

Anterior Compartment

**ANTERIOR
COMPARTMENT
PROXIMAL**
Transverse
FIG. 5.32

The patient should be supine with the knee flexed to 90 degrees and the sole of the foot resting on the examination table. By palpation, identify the tibial tuberosity and anterior border of the tibia. Place the probe transversely over the proximal part of the anterior compartment just below the inferior extent of the tibial tuberosity. Identify the hyperechoic anterolateral surface of the tibia and its dense acoustic shadow. Adjust the probe position until the fibula is in view at the lateral extent of the image. Locate the hyperechoic tibiofibular interosseous membrane spanning between the medial surface of the fibula and the anterolateral surface of the tibia in the deep part of the image. Tibialis anterior is the large muscle seen along the tibia and medial half of the interosseous membrane. Identify the extensor digitorum longus muscle between tibialis anterior and the hyperechoic anterior intermuscular septum, which spans between the medial surface of the fibula and the deep surface of the crural fascia. The fibularis longus muscle is partly in view lateral to the anterior intermuscular septum, in the lateral compartment. Toggle (tilt and fan) the probe face to locate the anterior tibial artery and deep fibular nerve in contact with the interosseous membrane deep to extensor digitorum longus. Part of the tibialis posterior muscle can be seen along the posterior surface of the interosseous membrane.

Figure 5.32   Transverse view of the proximal third of the anterior compartment of the leg.

Starting from the previous probe position, slide the probe distally along the anterior compartment to midleg (or just beyond midleg) keeping tibialis anterior, extensor digitorum longus, tibia, fibula, and tibiofibular interosseous membrane in view. While sliding the probe distally, passively flex and extend the big toe and watch for flashes of corresponding motion in the deep part of the compartment along the medial surface of the fibula and adjacent interosseous membrane, to identify the extensor hallucis longus muscle and to delineate its borders. Note the characteristic hyperechoic central tendon of tibialis anterior muscle in the midleg. The fibularis brevis muscle is partly in view lateral to flexor digitorum longus and along the lateral surface of the fibula. The anterior intermuscular septum separating fibularis brevis from extensor digitorum longus may be difficult to see because of anisotropy. Toggle (tilt and fan) the probe face to locate the anterior tibial artery and deep fibular nerve in the deep part of the image between extensor hallucis longus, tibialis anterior, and the tibiofibular interosseous membrane.

Lateral Compartment

The patient should be in lateral decubitus position with a small pillow/bolster between the knees and the knee flexed to 90 degrees. Locate the head and neck of the fibula by palpation and place the probe transversely (marker directed anteriorly) over the lateral aspect of the leg at the junction of the fibular head and neck. Identify the hyperechoic surface of the fibula and its acoustic shadow. Slide the probe superiorly and inferiorly a short distance and observe the change in profile from the larger ovoid head to the narrow neck. Adjust the probe position and toggle/tilt the probe face to identify the hyperechoic

Figure 5.33 Transverse view of the anterior compartment at midleg.

common fibular nerve as it courses obliquely across the neck of the fibula deep to the fibularis longus muscle. Identify the fibularis longus muscle with its rounded anterior and posterior edges. The hyperechoic anterior intermuscular septum is seen along the deep surface of the anterior part of fibularis longus, extending from the fibula to the deep (crural) fascia, separating the lateral and anterior compartments of the leg. The posterior intermuscular septum is seen along the deep surface of the posterior part of fibularis longus, extending from the fibula to the crural fascia, separating the lateral and posterior compartments.

LATERAL COMPARTMENT MIDLEG
Transverse
FIG. 5.35

Starting from the previous probe position, slide the probe distally along the lateral compartment to about midleg, keeping the fibularis longus muscle centered in the image. Fibularis longus begins to narrow in its lateral-medial dimension, and its connective tissue density increases as fibularis brevis muscle appears and enlarges along the lateral surface of the fibula, between the fibula and fibularis longus. Again, identify the anterior intermuscular septum separating the lateral and anterior compartments and the posterior intermuscular septum separating the lateral and posterior compartments.

LATERAL COMPARTMENT DISTAL THIRD OF LEG
Transverse
FIG. 5.36

Beginning from the previous probe position, slide the probe distally along the lateral compartment to the junction between the proximal and distal thirds of the leg, keeping fibularis longus and brevis centered in the image. Approaching the distal third of the leg, fibularis longus narrows to a tendinous band along the superficial surface of fibularis brevis. More distally, the tendinous band becomes an oval tendon posterior to the tendon of fibularis brevis. The anterior part of fibularis brevis muscle narrows to form an oval tendon at the posterior surface of the distal fibula, whereas the posterior muscular part persists as far as the posterior surface of the lateral malleolus. Identify the anterior intermuscular septum separating the lateral and anterior compartments and the posterior intermuscular septum separating the lateral and posterior compartments.

Figure 5.34 Transverse view of the lateral compartment of the leg at the level of the neck of the fibula.

Posterior Compartment

POSTERIOR COMPARTMENT MIDLEG
Transverse
FIG. 5.37

The patient should be prone with the ankles and feet over the end of the examination table. Place the probe transversely over the center of the posterior aspect of the leg at the inferior extent of the calf belly, at or just below midleg (probe marker directed laterally). Adjust the probe position as needed to identify the inferior extent of the medial and lateral heads of gastrocnemius and their intervening aponeurotic tendon overlying the soleus muscle and its tendinous superficial surface. Applying minimal pressure to the probe face, slide the probe superiorly and inferiorly while toggling/tilting the probe to identify the small saphenous vein and accompanying sural nerve within a compartment of the crural fascia superficial to the aponeurotic tendon between the heads of gastrocnemius. Adjust the probe position and tilt as needed to identify the rounded oblong contour of the soleus muscle. Deep to the medial aspect of soleus, between soleus and the deep muscles of the posterior compartment, identify the tibial nerve and posterior tibial vessels.

POSTERIOR COMPARTMENT MIDLEG
Longitudinal
FIG. 5.38

Starting from the previous probe position, slide the probe medially bringing the lower part of the medial head of gastrocnemius into the center of the image. Rotate the probe 90 degrees (marker side directed superiorly) into the longitudinal axis of the leg and adjust the probe position to bring the tapering distal end of the medial head of gastrocnemius into view. Deep to gastrocnemius, identify the soleus muscle and note the tendinous layer along its superficial surface. At the distal end of gastrocnemius, the gastrocnemius aponeurotic tendon joins the soleus tendon forming the

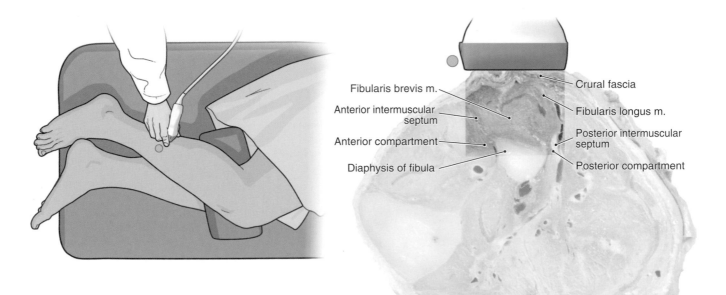

Fibularis brevis m.
Anterior intermuscular septum
Anterior compartment
Diaphysis of fibula

Crural fascia
Fibularis longus m.
Posterior intermuscular septum
Posterior compartment

Crural fascia
Fibularis longus m.
Fibularis brevis m.
Posterior intermuscular septum
Anterior intermuscular septum
Diaphysis of fibula
Anterior compartment
Posterior compartment

Figure 5.35 Transverse view of the lateral compartment muscles at midleg.

calcaneal tendon. Sliding distally in the same plane, the calcaneal tendon progressively thickens as tendon fibers from soleus are added to it. Deep to soleus identify the deep muscle layer of the posterior compartment. From medial to lateral, the deep muscles are flexor digitorum longus, tibialis posterior, and flexor hallucis longus. Tilt the probe face as needed to identify the hyperechoic posterior surface of the tibia and its acoustic shadow.

POSTERIOR COMPARTMENT CALCANEAL TENDON DISTAL LEG
Longitudinal
FIG. 5.39

By palpation, locate the calcaneal tendon in the distal leg. Place the probe over the tendon in its longitudinal axis 4 to 6 cm above the heel (marker directed superiorly). Note the hyperechoic fibrillar appearance of the thick calcaneal tendon. Adjust the probe position superiorly/inferiorly along the tendon until the tapering inferior end of soleus can be clearly seen. Look for the numerous parallel hyperechoic lines of connective tissue (perimysium) within soleus to help distinguish the distal end of soleus from Kager's fat pad beyond (the hyperechoic connective tissue lines in the fat pad are much less organized). The triangular profile of Kager's fat pad is seen deep to the calcaneal tendon with its apex projecting between the distal end of soleus and the deep group of muscles. Flexor hallucis longus is the main muscle of the deep group seen in this position. Look for the hyperechoic posterior surface of the tibia, which curves posteriorly into a rounded hump at its distal end, referred to clinically as the posterior malleolus.

Figure 5.36 Transverse view of the lateral compartment in the distal third of the leg.

CLINICAL APPLICATIONS

US examination is useful for the evaluation of muscle and tendon injuries, including tendinosis/tendonitis and partial or complete tears of the gastrocnemius and/or soleus muscles and their aponeurotic tendons, the calcaneal tendon, and the ankle extensor (dorsiflexor) tendons (tibialis anterior, extensor digitorum longus, and extensor hallucis longus). Most injuries of the fibularis tendons occur at the ankle joint.

US measurement of anterior compartment thickness before and after a period of exertion is being increasingly used in the diagnosis of chronic exertional compartment syndrome.

US examination and measurement may be used in the evaluation of entrapment/compression of the common fibular nerve in its course along the fibular head and neck, the superficial fibular nerve as it pierces the deep fascia in the distal leg, the deep fibular nerve in its course

through the anterior compartment (by osteophytes, space-occupying lesions, or scar tissue), the sural nerve where it pierces deep fascia in the distal leg, and the tibial nerve where it passes under the tendinous arch of the soleus muscle origin into the posterior leg compartment.

US-guided nerve blocks are used in a variety of surgeries involving the distal leg, ankle, and foot, including blocks of the tibial nerve, common fibular nerve, superficial fibular nerve, deep fibular nerve, saphenous nerve, and sural nerve. US examination is used to evaluate the posterior tibial and fibular veins when deep vein thrombosis is suspected. The anterior tibial veins are much less commonly involved in deep vein thrombosis and so are not routinely scanned. In the evaluation of peripheral artery disease, arteries that are included in Doppler US studies of the leg include the popliteal, posterior tibial, fibular, and anterior tibial.

Figure 5.37 Transverse view of the posterior compartment at midleg, including the small saphenous vein and sural nerve.

Medial
gastrocnemius m.

Gastrocnemius
aponeurosis

Aponeurotic tendon
of soleus

Calcaneal
tendon

Soleus m.

Flexor
digitorum
longus m.

Tibia

Gastrocnemius
aponeurosis

Medial gastrocnemius m.

Aponeurotic
tendon of soleus

Calcaneal
tendon

Soleus m.

Flexor digitorum longus m.

Tibia

Figure 5.38 Longitudinal (parasagittal) view of the medial aspect of the posterior compartment
at midleg.

Figure 5.39 Longitudinal view of the posterior compartment in the distal leg, including the calcaneal tendon, the distal end of soleus, and Kager's fat pad.

Ankle and Foot

Review of the Anatomy

Bones

The bones of the foot include 7 tarsal bones, 5 metatarsals, and 3 phalanges for each toe except the big toe, which has only 2 phalanges.

Tarsal Bones

Talus

The main part of the talus is referred to as the body. The trochlea of the talus, which articulates with the tibia and fibula to form the ankle joint, projects superiorly from the body. A small lateral process projects laterally from the body over the lateral surface of calcaneus. The posterior process of the talus projects posteriorly from the body and has 2 rounded projections, the medial and lateral tubercles, with a groove between them for the tendon of flexor hallucis longus. A short neck projects anteriorly from the body to the rounded head at the anterior surface of the talus, which articulates with the navicular bone. The talus sits on top of and is supported by the calcaneus.

Calcaneus

The calcaneus is the largest of the tarsal bones. The superior surface of calcaneus has 3 articular facets for the talus forming the subtalar joint. Part of the calcaneus projects behind the ankle joint to form the heel. The posterior surface is semicircular with a facet for insertion of the calcaneal tendon posteriorly and expands below to the calcaneal tuberosity at the plantar surface of the heel. At its anterior aspect the calcaneal tuberosity has 2 projections separated by a shallow groove, the medial and lateral processes. The plantar aponeurosis attaches to the larger medial process and intervening groove.

A thick bony shelf, the sustentaculum tali, projects medially from the upper anterior part of the calcaneus. Its superior surface supports and articulates with the talus at the junction of the head and neck, and there is a groove for the tendon of flexor hallucis longus along its undersurface.

The tendons of fibularis longus and brevis course across the lateral surface of calcaneus and are separated by a small projection, the fibular trochlea, as they pass through separate compartments of the inferior fibular retinaculum.

The anterior surface of the calcaneus articulates with the cuboid bone.

Other Tarsal Bones

The navicular bone articulates posteriorly with the head of the talus and anteriorly with the medial, intermediate, and lateral cuneiform bones, which articulate anteriorly with the bases of metatarsal bones I, II, and III, respectively. The cuboid bone articulates posteriorly with calcaneus, medially with the medial cuneiform bone, and anteriorly with the bases of metatarsals IV and V. There is a groove along the plantar surface of the cuboid bone for the tendon of fibularis longus.

Metatarsals

The metatarsal bones, numbered I through V from medial to lateral, have bases proximally and heads distally, joined by their bodies. The metatarsal heads articulate proximally with the medial, intermediate, and lateral cuneiform bones (I, II, and III, respectively) and the cuboid bone (IV and V), as well as with one another. There is a prominent posterolateral projection, the tubercle, from the base of metatarsal V, which serves as a site of attachment for the tendon of fibularis brevis. The heads of the metatarsals articulate with the proximal phalanges of the toes.

Ankle Joint

The ankle joint is formed between the distal ends of the leg bones, the tibia and fibula, and the talus. The expanded distal end of the tibia forms the superior and medial (medial malleolus) surfaces of the bony arch of the ankle joint, often referred to clinically as the ankle *mortise*. The lateral malleolus of the fibula forms the lateral surface of the ankle joint arch or mortise. The cylindrical trochlea of the talus projects superiorly from the body of the talus into the arch formed by the tibia and fibula. A synovial membrane attached along the margins of the articular surfaces of the tibia, fibula, and trochlea of the talus lines the joint. The synovial membrane is in turn covered by a fibrous capsule with similar bony attachments. The ankle joint is stabilized by medial and lateral collateral ligament complexes, which also reinforce the joint capsule medially and laterally. The capsule is lax anteriorly and posteriorly (the anterior and posterior recesses) where it is not reinforced by ligaments.

A number of tendons cross the ankle joint to reach their attachments in the foot. The tendons of tibialis posterior, flexor digitorum longus, and flexor hallucis longus cross the ankle joint posteromedially through the tarsal tunnel. The calcaneal tendon crosses the joint posteriorly. The tendons of fibularis longus and brevis cross the ankle joint posterolaterally along the posterior surface of the lateral malleolus. The tendons of tibialis anterior, extensor hallucis longus, and extensor digitorum longus cross the joint anteriorly.

Ligaments

Tibiofibular Ligaments

The tibia and fibula are joined by the tibiofibular interosseous membrane. Reinforcing the interosseous membrane just above the ankle joint, the distal tibia and fibula are joined by anterior and posterior tibiofibular ligaments.

Fibular Collateral Ligament Complex

The anterior talofibular, posterior talofibular, and calcaneofibular ligaments are the 3 components of the fibular collateral ligament of the ankle. The lateral ligaments of the ankle are not as strong as the medial (tibial) ligaments. The anterior talofibular ligament, the weakest and most commonly injured of the lateral ligaments, spans between the anterior edge of the lateral malleolus and the dorsal aspect of the neck of the talus. The posterior talofibular ligament spans between the posterior nonarticular part of the medial surface of the lateral malleolus and the lateral tubercle of the posterior process of the talus. The calcaneofibular ligament attaches between the tip of the lateral malleolus and a small tubercle on the posterolateral surface of the calcaneus just behind the ankle joint. The tendons of fibularis brevis and longus cross over the ligament as they turn anteriorly from the posterior surface of the lateral malleolus.

Tibial Collateral Ligament Complex (Deltoid Ligament)

Referred to collectively as the **deltoid ligament**, the medial ligament complex of the ankle has 4 named parts: the anterior tibiotalar ligament, the tibionavicular ligament, the tibiocalcaneal ligament, and the posterior tibiotalar ligament. The components of the deltoid ligament are larger and stronger than the lateral ankle ligaments.

The tibionavicular ligament attaches between the anterior inferior surface of the medial malleolus to the medial surface of the navicular bone and the superior/medial margin of the plantar calcaneonavicular (spring) ligament just behind the navicular. The anterior tibiotalar ligament, deep to the tibionavicular ligament, attaches between the anterior inferior edge of the medial malleolus and the medial surface of the talus from the head to the body. The tibiocalcaneal ligament, nearly vertical, spans between the inferior edge of the medial malleolus and the sustentaculum tali of calcaneus. The posterior tibiotalar ligament attaches between the posterior inferior edge of the medial malleolus and the medial surface of the talus from the medial tubercle of the posterior process to the body. Most of the superficial surface of the deltoid ligament is crossed by the tendons of tibialis posterior and flexor digitorum longus in their course through and just beyond the tarsal tunnel.

Tendons, Nerves, and Arteries Crossing the Ankle

Anterior Compartment of the Leg

The anterior compartment muscles, innervated by the deep fibular nerve, are tibialis anterior, extensor hallucis longus, extensor digitorum longus, and fibularis tertius. Their tendons cross the anterior aspect of the ankle joint deep to superior and inferior extensor retinacula onto the dorsum of the foot. The deep fibular nerve and anterior tibial vessels descend through the anterior compartment to cross the ankle joint anteriorly along with the tendons of the anterior compartment muscles.

Anterior Compartment Tendons

Tibialis anterior becomes tendinous in the distal third of the leg, crosses the ankle joint as the most medial of the anterior compartment tendons, and turns under the medial side of the foot to insert at the base of the first metatarsal and adjacent plantar surface of the medial cuneiform bone.

Extensor hallucis longus is covered at its origin by tibialis anterior medially and by extensor digitorum longus laterally. Its tendon emerges between the 2 in the distal third of the leg to cross the ankle joint between their tendons, continuing across the dorsum of the foot to insert onto the dorsal surface of the base of the distal phalanx of the great toe.

The tendon of extensor digitorum longus forms in the distal leg and crosses the ankle joint lateral to the tendon of extensor hallucis longus. On the dorsum of the foot, the tendon divides into 4 slips that insert into the extensor expansions of the lateral toes.

Dorsalis Pedis Artery

The dorsalis pedis artery (usually the continuation of the anterior tibial artery beyond the ankle joint) crosses the ankle just lateral to the tendon of extensor hallucis longus and continues alongside the tendon onto the dorsum of the foot where it has dorsal metatarsal branches and a deep plantar branch, which anastomoses with the deep plantar arterial arch.

Deep Fibular Nerve

The deep fibular nerve is lateral to the anterior tibial artery as it crosses the ankle onto the dorsum of the foot. Just after crossing the ankle it gives a motor branch to extensor digitorum brevis and continues distally, becoming cutaneous in the web space between the great and second toes.

Lateral Compartment of the Leg

The 2 lateral compartment muscles, fibularis longus and brevis, are innervated by the superficial fibular nerve. Their tendons cross the ankle joint along the posterior surface of the lateral malleolus.

Lateral Compartment Tendons

Fibularis longus becomes tendinous about midleg and descends along the superficial surface of fibularis brevis and more distally along the posterior surface of the distal fibula and lateral malleolus where it is immediately lateral to the tendon of fibularis brevis. Fibularis brevis becomes tendinous as it descends along the posterior surface of the distal fibula and lateral malleolus.

At the posterior edge of the tip of the lateral malleolus, both tendons cross under the small superior fibular retinaculum and then over the calcaneofibular ligament as they begin to turn anteriorly across the lateral surface of calcaneus. A short distance anteriorly, they cross through separate compartments of the small inferior fibular retinaculum where they are separated by the fibular trochlea of calcaneus. The tendon of fibularis brevis lies above the trochlea and the tendon of fibularis longus lies below it.

Beyond the fibular trochlea the tendon of fibularis brevis continues anteriorly along the lateral surface of calcaneus and the lateral surface of the cuboid bone to insert at the tubercle of the base of the fifth metacarpal.

The tendon of fibularis longus continues anteriorly across the lateral surface of calcaneus, curving deeply at the anterior aspect of calcaneus to approach the cuboid bone where it enters a groove along its plantar surface. The tendon turns medially in the groove and courses obliquely across the plantar foot to attach at the base of the first metatarsal and adjacent medial cuneiform bone. A sesamoid bone may be present adjacent to the base of the fifth metatarsal where the tendon turns into the groove in the cuboid bone.

Superficial Fibular Nerve

The superficial fibular nerve descends in the lateral compartment, which it supplies, deep to fibularis longus and then emerges between fibularis brevis and extensor digitorum longus in the distal third of the leg. It pierces the deep fascia a variable distance above the lateral malleolus and divides into its terminal branches, the medial and intermediate dorsal cutaneous nerves. The medial dorsal cutaneous branch supplies the medial aspect of the dorsum of the foot and proximal part of the great toe. The intermediate dorsal cutaneous nerve supplies most of the remainder of the dorsum of the foot and proximal parts of the second through fifth toes.

Posterior Compartment of the Leg

The posterior compartment muscles, innervated by the tibial nerve, are arranged in superficial and deep layers.

Superficial Layer

The muscles of the superficial group include the medial and lateral heads of gastrocnemius, soleus, and the small plantaris muscle. The 2 heads of gastrocnemius converge at the inferior extent of the popliteal fossa and taper to a broad flattened tendinous band (gastrocnemius aponeurosis) about midleg. Tendinous fibers begin to appear along the central posterior part of soleus muscle in the midcalf. The tendon of soleus fuses with the overlying tendon of gastrocnemius to complete the formation of the calcaneal tendon in the distal third of the leg.

The calcaneal tendon continues distally, superficial to Kager's fat pad, to insert onto the midportion of the posterior surface of calcaneus.

Kager's Fat Pad and Retrocalcaneal Bursa

Kager's fat pad is located in the distal leg and posterior to the ankle joint. The fat pad has a triangular shape, with the base formed by the superior cortical surface of calcaneus, the anterior border formed by flexor hallucis longus muscle and tendon, and the posterior border formed by the anterior (deep) surface of the calcaneal tendon. The apex of the triangle extends superiorly between the distal fibers of soleus and the muscles of the deep group. The retrocalcaneal bursa, which intervenes between the upper posterior surface of calcaneus and the calcaneal tendon, is located at the posterior inferior corner of the triangle. The bursa may not be seen unless it is inflamed.

Deep Layer

The muscles of the deep group include popliteus, tibialis posterior, flexor digitorum longus, and flexor hallucis longus. Popliteus is a short muscle related to the knee joint previously discussed along with structures of the knee. The tendons tibialis posterior, flexor digitorum longus, and flexor hallucis longus cross the medial side of the ankle joint through the tarsal tunnel to enter the plantar aspect of the foot.

Tarsal Tunnel

The tarsal tunnel is a fibro-osseous tunnel consisting of a shallow depression along the posterior surface of the medial malleolus, the medial surface of the posterior process and body of the talus, and the medial surface of calcaneus, spanned by the flexor retinaculum. The flexor retinaculum is a band of fibrous connective tissue attached anteriorly along the inferior margin of the medial malleolus and posteriorly to the medial surface of calcaneus. Fibrous septae from the deep surface of the retinaculum form separate compartments within the tarsal tunnel for the tendons of the deep posterior compartment muscles and for the neurovascular bundle consisting of the posterior tibial vessels and the tibial nerve.

In the distal leg, the tendon of flexor digitorum longus crosses the tendon of tibialis posterior superficially from anterior to posterior, so that in the tarsal tunnel, the tibialis posterior tendon lies along the posterior surface of the medial malleolus immediately anterior to the flexor digitorum longus tendon. The tendon of flexor hallucis longus enters the tarsal tunnel in a groove between the medial and lateral tubercles of the posterior process of the talus and so is separated from the tendons of tibialis posterior and flexor digitorum longus. Beyond the groove in the posterior process of talus, the flexor hallucis longus tendon enters a groove along the inferior surface of the sustentaculum tali of calcaneus. The neurovascular bundle is located in the space between the tendon of flexor digitorum longus anteriorly and the tendon of flexor hallucis longus posteriorly. The vessels, the posterior tibial artery and 2 or 3 accompanying veins are just behind the tendon of flexor digitorum longus with the tibial nerve just posterior to the vessels. Within the tunnel, the neurovascular bundle is slightly anterior and superficial (medial) to the tendon of flexor hallucis longus.

Tendons and Insertions

All 3 tendons turn anteriorly in the tunnel, exiting the tunnel deep to abductor hallucis muscle and curving under the medial aspect of the foot to reach their attachments.

The tendon of tibialis posterior fans out to attach to the plantar surfaces of the navicular bone and adjacent cuneiform bones along the medial aspect of the foot. The tendon of flexor hallucis longus continues distally, inserting at the plantar surface of the base of the distal phalanx of the great toe. The tendon of flexor digitorum longus crosses under (inferior or superficial to) the flexor hallucis longus tendon and divides into 4 slips that insert onto the plantar surfaces of the bases of the distal phalanges of the lateral toes.

Posterior Tibial Artery

In the distal part of the tarsal tunnel, or just after exiting the tunnel, the posterior tibial artery and its accompanying veins divide into 3 branches: medial calcaneal, lateral plantar, and medial plantar. The lateral plantar artery crosses to the lateral side of the foot deep to flexor digitorum brevis, a superficial intrinsic muscle of the foot, and then curves medially to form the deep plantar arterial arch. The medial plantar artery continues distally along the medial aspect of the foot.

Tibial Nerve

The tibial nerve has a similar course and branching pattern as the posterior tibial artery. A medial calcaneal branch accompanies the similarly named artery onto the plantar surface of the posterior part of calcaneus, and lateral medial and plantar nerves accompany the similarly named arteries. The large lateral plantar nerve provides cutaneous supply to most of the plantar aspect of the foot and lateral 3½ toes and motor supply to most of the intrinsic muscles of the foot. The smaller medial plantar nerve provides cutaneous innervation to the medial aspect of the plantar foot and medial 1½ toes and motor innervation to 4 intrinsic muscles of the foot not supplied by the lateral plantar nerve.

Plantar Aponeurosis

The plantar aponeurosis is a distinct thickened band of deep fascia that attaches posteriorly to the periosteum of the medial process of the calcaneal tubercle and extends anteriorly along the central part of the sole of the foot, over the superficial surface of flexor digitorum brevis muscle. At about midfoot the aponeurosis begins to expand medially and laterally, dividing into separate bands for each of the toes, which attach to the metatarsophalangeal joint capsules and associated ligaments.

Technique

Anterior Aspect of the Ankle Joint

Anterior Compartment Tendons

ANTERIOR COMPARTMENT TENDONS ANKLE JOINT
Transverse
FIG. 5.40

The patient should be supine with the knee flexed to 90 degrees and the sole of the foot resting on the examination table. Place the probe transversely over the distal part of the anterior compartment a few centimeters above the medial and lateral malleoli. In the distal leg, the muscles of the anterior compartment become progressively smaller as their tendinous components enlarge and become more evident. Tilt/toggle the probe face to identify the hyperechoic tendons (and remaining muscle tissue) of tibialis anterior, extensor hallucis longus, and extensor digitorum longus.

Slide the probe distally, keeping the tendons in view, to a position between the medial and lateral malleoli. Look for the shallow concave hyperechoic surface of the trochlea of the talus covered by an anechoic layer of hyaline cartilage, occupying most or all of the deep part of the image. The joint capsule and synovial lining of the anterior recess of the ankle joint can be seen superficial to the trochlea of the talus. Superficial to the joint capsule, identify the tibialis anterior tendon at the medial aspect of the image, toggling the probe face as needed to minimize anisotropy. A short distance lateral to the tibialis anterior tendon, identify the tendon/myotendinous junction of extensor hallucis longus. Lateral to extensor hallucis longus, identify the tendon/myotendinous junction of extensor digitorum longus. Deep to the lateral edge of extensor hallucis longus (toggling the probe face as needed), identify the deep fibular nerve and anterior tibial artery.

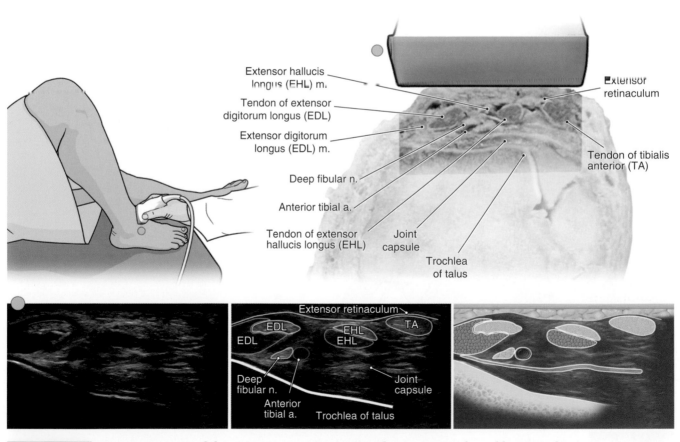

Extensor hallucis longus (EHL) m.
Tendon of extensor digitorum longus (EDL)
Extensor digitorum longus (EDL) m.
Deep fibular n.
Anterior tibial a.
Tendon of extensor hallucis longus (EHL)
Extensor retinaculum
Tendon of tibialis anterior (TA)
Joint capsule
Trochlea of talus

Extensor retinaculum
EDL
EDL
EHL
EHL
TA
Deep fibular n.
Anterior tibial a.
Joint capsule
Trochlea of talus

Figure 5.40 Transverse view of the anterior compartment tendons crossing the ankle joint, along with the deep fibular nerve and anterior tibial artery.

Anterior Tibiofibular Ligament

ANTERIOR TIBIOFIBULAR LIGAMENT
Longitudinal
FIG. 5.41

The patient should be supine with the knee flexed to 90 degrees and the sole of the foot resting on the examination table. Place the probe transversely over the anterolateral aspect of the leg, with marker side of the probe over the anterior edge of the lateral malleolus about 1 cm above the tip of the malleolus. Identify the hyperechoic surface and acoustic shadow of the lateral malleolus. Keeping the marker side of the probe anchored in position, rotate the heel (nonmarker side) of the probe superiorly so that it comes to lie about 2 cm higher on the leg than the marker side. This brings the probe face approximately parallel to the longitudinal axis of the anterior tibiofibular ligament. Look for the bony profile of the distal tibia and the distal tibiofibular joint to come into view. Adjust the probe position and tilt to identify the fibrillar appearance of anterior tibiofibular ligament as it spans the tibiofibular joint between the anterior surfaces of the lateral malleolus and lateral aspect of the distal tibia. Internal rotation of the foot will place tension on the ligament.

Anterior Talofibular Ligament

ANTERIOR TALOFIBULAR LIGAMENT
Longitudinal
FIG. 5.42

The patient should be supine with the knee flexed to 90 degrees and the sole of the foot resting on the examination table. Alternatively, the patient can be positioned in lateral decubitus with the knee slightly flexed and a small bolster placed under the medial side of the ankle to allow the examiner to passively plantarflex and invert the foot, placing tension on the ligament. Starting with the probe in the position described earlier to image the anterior tibiofibular ligament, slide the probe slightly inferiorly so that the marker side of the probe is over the anterior surface of the tip of the lateral malleolus and rotate the heel of the probe downward approximately 90 degrees across the anterior aspect of the ankle joint (the anterior tibiofibular and anterior talofibular ligaments are nearly at right angles to one another). During the rotation, the probe sweeps across the articular surface of the trochlea of the talus and onto the neck of the talus. Adjust the probe position and tilt until you can identify the hyperechoic fibrillar appearance of the anterior talofibular ligament spanning between the anterior edge of the tip of the lateral malleolus and the neck of the talus.

Figure 5.41 Longitudinal view of the anterior tibiofibular ligament.

Lateral Aspect of the Ankle Joint

Tendons of Fibularis Longus and Brevis

FIBULARIS LONGUS TENDON
FIBULARIS BREVIS TENDON
LATERAL MALLEOLUS
Transverse
FIG. 5.43

The patient should be in lateral decubitus position with a small pillow or bolster between the slightly flexed knees. Place the probe face transverse to the long axis of the leg with the marker side of the probe at the posterolateral aspect of the superior part of the lateral malleolus. Adjust the probe position and tilt/fan the probe face, minimizing anisotropy, to identify the tendon of fibularis longus. Immediately posteromedial to the fibularis longus tendon, the tendon of fibularis brevis is incompletely formed at this level and more difficult to definitively identify. A small ovoid component of fibularis brevis muscle is seen along the posterior aspect of the forming tendon. Keeping the lateral malleolus and fibularis tendons in view, slide the probe posteriorly as needed, while minimizing probe face pressure, to locate the small saphenous vein in superficial fascia a short distance behind the lateral malleolus.

Calcaneofibular Ligament

CALCANEOFIBULAR LIGAMENT
Longitudinal
FIG. 5.44

With the patient in lateral decubitus position as described earlier, dorsiflex the foot to place tension on the calcaneofibular ligament and to bring it into alignment with the long axis of the fibula. Place the marker side of the probe at the tip of the lateral malleolus with the heel of the probe positioned slightly posteriorly, bringing the probe face into alignment with the longitudinal axis of the calcaneofibular ligament. Adjust the probe position and tilt to identify the tendons of fibularis longus and brevis, and immediately deep to the tendons, the hyperechoic fibrillar calcaneofibular ligament spanning from the medial surface of the lateral malleolus (hidden in acoustic shadow) to the lateral surface of the posterior part of calcaneus a short distance below the tip of the malleolus.

Fibularis Brevis Tendon

FIBULARIS BREVIS TENDON INSERTION
Longitudinal
FIG. 5.45

The patient should be in lateral decubitus position with a small pillow or bolster between the slightly flexed knees. Locate the

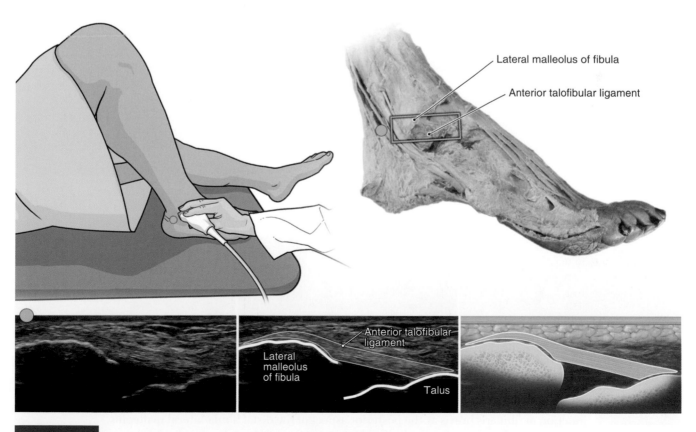

Lateral malleolus of fibula

Anterior talofibular ligament

Anterior talofibular ligament

Lateral malleolus of fibula

Talus

Figure 5.42   Longitudinal view of the anterior talofibular ligament.

tubercle of the base of the fifth metatarsal by palpation. Ask the patient to evert the foot. The tendon of fibularis brevis is usually visible from just below and anterior to the tip of the lateral malleolus to its insertion at the tubercle of the fifth metatarsal base. With the muscles around the ankle again relaxed, position the probe along the longitudinal axis of the tendon with the marker side directed toward the anterior aspect of the tip of the lateral malleolus and the heel over the posterior aspect of the tubercle of the fifth metatarsal base. Identify the rounded hyperechoic surface and acoustic shadow of the tubercle. Adjust the probe position until the hyperechoic fibrillar appearance of the fibularis brevis tendon can be seen along with its insertion onto the tubercle. Proximal to its insertion, the tendon passes over the anterior part of the lateral surface of calcaneus and the lateral surface of the cuboid bone.

Fibularis Longus Tendon

FIBULARIS LONGUS TENDON CALCANEUS
Longitudinal
FIG. 5.46

With the patient in lateral decubitus position as described earlier, position the probe along a line interconnecting the tip of the lateral malleolus and a point about 1 cm posterior to the tubercle of the base of the fifth metatarsal. Adjust the probe position until the hyperechoic fibrillar appearance of the fibularis longus tendon can be identified. Identify the lateral surface of calcaneus deep to the tendon. As needed, slide the probe distally along the tendon until it can be seen curving toward the plantar surface of the foot along the anterior part of calcaneus approaching the cuboid bone (the fibrillar appearance of the tendon disappears because of anisotropy).

Tendon of fibularis longus (FL)
Tendon of fibularis brevis
Lateral malleolus of fibula
Small saphenous v.

FL
Small saphenous v.
Lateral malleolus of fibula
Tendon of fibularis brevis

Figure 5.43 Transverse view of the tendon of fibularis longus and the tendon/myotendinous junction of fibularis brevis at the posterior aspect of the distal fibula/lateral malleolus.

Medial Aspect of the Ankle Joint

Tarsal Tunnel and Contents

**TARSAL TUNNEL
MEDIAL MALLEOLUS**
Transverse
FIG. 5.47

The patient should be supine with the knee slightly flexed and the thigh externally rotated ("frog-leg" position). A small pillow or bolster should be placed under the lateral aspect of the ankle to allow for eversion of the foot, to minimize the concavity of the tarsal tunnel. Place the marker side of the probe along the inferior edge of the medial malleolus with the probe face angled toward the heel. Adjust the probe position and tilt to identify the tendon of tibialis posterior along the medial malleolus. Immediately posterior (and slightly deep/medial) to the tibialis posterior tendon, identify the tendon of flexor digitorum longus (adjusting the probe position slightly and fanning/tilting the probe face as needed to minimize anisotropy). Keeping the tendons of tibialis posterior and flexor digitorum longus in view, adjust the probe position and tilt until the tendon of flexor hallucis longus can be

identified in a groove along the posterior process of the talus. Owing to anisotropy, the flexor hallucis longus tendon can be somewhat difficult to identify. Locating the rounded profile of the medial tubercle of the posterior process of the talus is often helpful in identifying the position of the flexor hallucis longus tendon. Immediately deep to the hyperechoic flexor retinaculum, the posterior tibial vessels and tibial nerve are seen posterior to the tendon of flexor digitorum longus.

Tibiocalcaneal Ligament

**TIBIOCALCANEAL
LIGAMENT**
Longitudinal
FIG. 5.48

Starting from the tarsal tunnel view described earlier, rotate the heel (nonmarker side) of the probe anteriorly while keeping the tendon of flexor hallucis longus in view. The marker end of the probe should move slightly anteriorly while rotating the nonmarker end. Slowly rotate the probe until the tendon disappears under a prominent shelf of bone, the sustentaculum tali of calcaneus. Another bony prominence, the medial surface of the body

Tendon of fibularis longus (FL)

Lateral malleolus of fibula

Tendon of fibularis brevis (FB)

Calcaneofibular ligament

Calcaneus (posterolateral surface)

Lateral malleolus of fibula

FL

FB

Calcaneofibular ligament

Calcaneus

Figure 5.44 Longitudinal view of the calcaneofibular ligament. The tendons of fibularis longus and brevis cross over the ligament as they turn under the tip of the lateral malleolus.

139

of the talus, should come into view between the medial malleolus and the sustentaculum tali. These 2 medial bony prominences have a somewhat similar appearance, but observing the course of the tendon of flexor hallucis longus helps to definitively identify the sustentaculum tali. At this point, the probe should have a nearly vertical alignment along the long axis of the limb, with the nonmarker end of the probe directed slightly posteriorly. Identify the medial malleolus, the medial surface of the body of the talus, and the sustentaculum tali of calcaneus. Adjust the probe position and tilt/fan the face to identify the tendon of tibialis posterior. The tendon profile is elongated in this position, as the tendon is oblique to the probe orientation. Owing to anisotropy the tendon may appear hypoechoic. Attempt to identify the tendon of flexor digitorum longus (also oblique to the probe orientation) inferior to the tibialis posterior tendon and superficial to the medial edge of the sustentaculum tali. The tendons are seen in this position in the distal (anterior) end of the tarsal tunnel, where they are located between the flexor retinaculum superficially and the tibiocalcaneal ligament on their deep surfaces. Carefully adjust the probe position and tilt as needed, and passively evert the foot to place tension on the tibiocalcaneal ligament,

so that its fibrillar appearance can be seen. The ligament spans between the medial surface and inferior margin of the medial malleolus to the superior surface of the sustentaculum tali.

Posterior Aspect of the Ankle Joint

CALCANEAL TENDON INSERTION
Longitudinal
FIG. 5.49

The patient should be prone with the ankles and feet over the end of the examination table. By palpation, locate the calcaneal tendon in the distal leg. Place the probe over the tendon in its longitudinal axis just above the heel (marker directed superiorly). Note the hyperechoic fibrillar appearance of the thick calcaneal tendon. With the probe face centered along the longitudinal axis of the calcaneal tendon, slide the probe distally until the tapered distal end of the tendon can be seen at its insertion onto the posterior surface of calcaneus. Identify the hyperechoic posterior surface of calcaneus and its dense acoustic shadow. Deep to the calcaneal tendon along the posterior superior margin of calcaneus, the base of the

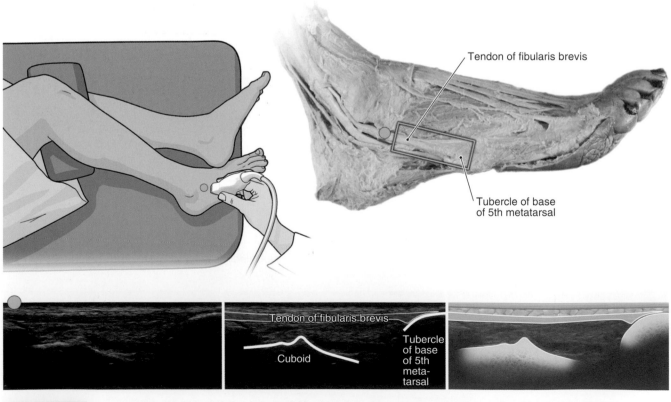

Tendon of fibularis brevis

Tubercle of base of 5th metatarsal

Tendon of fibularis brevis

Cuboid

Tubercle of base of 5th metatarsal

Figure 5.45 Longitudinal view of the tendon of fibularis brevis crossing over the cuboid bone to its insertion at the tubercle of the base of the fifth metatarsal.

triangular profile of Kager's fat pad can be seen. The retrocalcaneal bursa is located between the calcaneal tendon and the upper posterior surface of calcaneus but may not be well seen unless it is inflamed.

Plantar Aponeurosis

PLANTAR APONEUROSIS
Longitudinal
FIG. 5.50

The patient should be prone with the ankles and feet over the end of the examination table. Place the probe over the plantar surface of the heel, oriented along the long axis of the foot, with the marker side directed posteriorly. Identify the hyperechoic surface and dense acoustic shadow of the calcaneal tuberosity. Slide the probe face medially and laterally to identify the medial process of the tuberosity. Tilt/fan the probe face until the fibrillar appearance of the thick (3-5 mm) plantar aponeurosis can be identified as it attaches to the periosteum over the medial process and then extends anteriorly along the superficial surface of flexor digitorum brevis muscle. Because of the density of overlying tissues, the image gain may need to be increased to adequately image the aponeurosis and muscle.

CLINICAL APPLICATIONS

US examination is useful for the evaluation of muscle and tendon injuries, including tendinosis/tendonitis and partial or complete tendon tears. Examples of ankle tendon injuries that are routinely examined using US include the calcaneal tendon and the fibularis longus and brevis tendons. Injuries of the ankle extensor tendons and deep posterior compartment tendons are less common, but they do occur and may be underdiagnosed.

Calcaneal tendon rupture tends to occur in older men during recreational activities, of, e.g., "week-end warriors." The tendons of fibularis longus and/or brevis may subluxate owing to tearing of the superior fibular retinaculum in association with inversion ankle sprain injuries. This leads to snapping lateral ankle pain and may progress to tendinosis/tendonitis or fraying and partial or complete rupture of a fibularis tendon, most commonly fibularis brevis at the posterior surface of the lateral malleolus.

The medial and lateral ligaments of the ankle joint are stretched and partially or completely torn in inversion/eversion ankle sprains. The anterior talofibular ligament is the most commonly involved lateral ligament in inversion ankle injuries, followed by the calcaneofibular ligament. The medial (deltoid) ankle ligaments may be torn in association with injuries involving foot eversion or inversion with external rotation, but because of the strength of the medial (deltoid) ligaments, avulsion fractures of the medial malleolus are more common.

Sometimes injury to the anterior tibiofibular ligament is referred to as high ankle sprain, and the ligament can be torn in association with a variety of ankle sprain injuries (and ankle fractures), especially those that involve forceful external rotation of the inverted or everted foot.

US examination is used in the diagnosis of Morton's neuroma, an enlargement (perineural fibroma) of a common digital plantar nerve, usually in the space between the third and fourth metatarsal heads, leading to entrapment and pain or numbness. US examination and measurement may be used in the evaluation of entrapment or compression of the tibial nerve in its course through the tarsal tunnel.

US guidance can be used in ankle blocks (tibial nerve, sural nerve, saphenous nerve, superficial fibular nerve, and deep fibular nerve) for surgical procedures in the foot.

In the evaluation of peripheral artery disease, arteries that are included in Doppler US studies of the ankle and foot include the dorsalis pedis and posterior tibial arteries.

Plantar fasciitis is a painful condition related to overuse and repetitive stress of the plantar aponeurosis, resulting in tearing and disruption of the normal collagen fiber organization. US is useful for detecting localized changes in organization and thickness of the plantar aponeurosis, for detecting calcified areas, and in some cases, for guiding steroid injections.

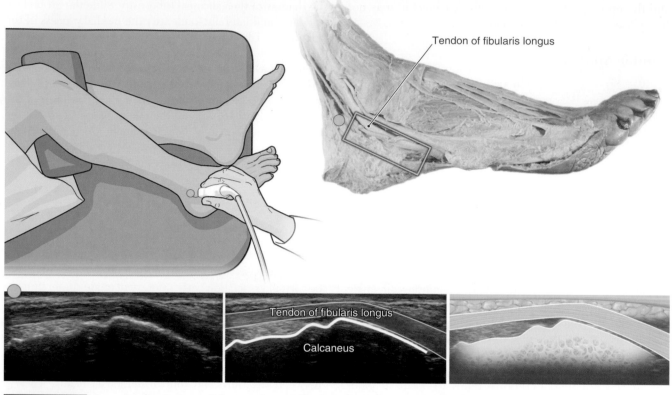

Figure 5.46 Longitudinal view of the tendon of fibularis longus crossing the lateral surface of calcaneus.

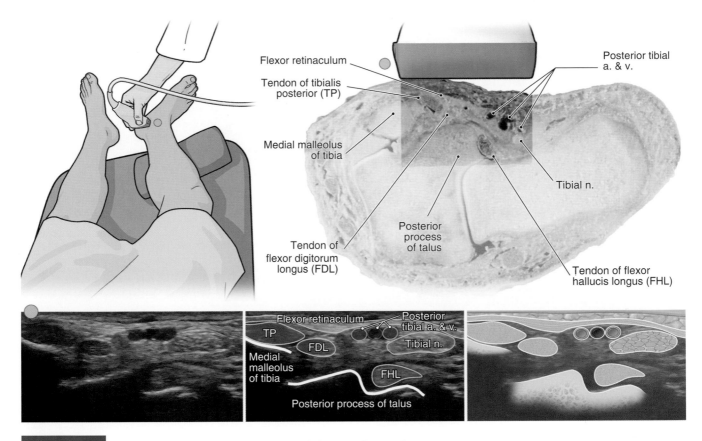

Figure 5.47 Transverse view of the contents of the tarsal tunnel.

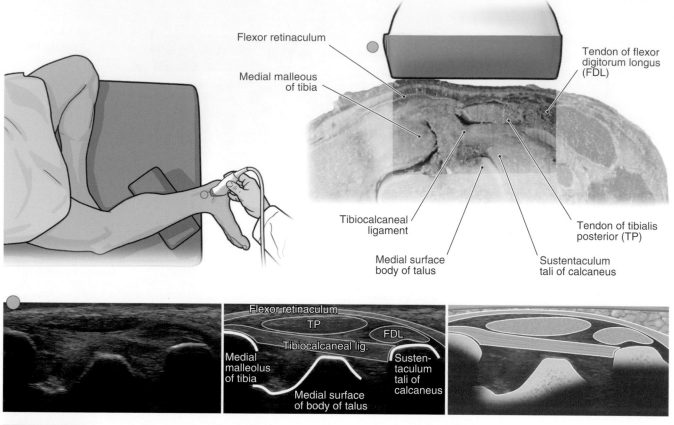

Figure 5.48 Longitudinal view of the tibiocalcaneal ligament (of the deltoid ligament complex) in the floor of the tarsal tunnel.

Calcaneal
tendon

Kager's fat pad

Retrocalcaneal bursa

Calcaneus

Calcaneal tendon

Calcaneus

Kager's
fat pad

Retrocalcaneal
bursa

Figure 5.49 Longitudinal view of the calcaneal tendon at its insertion onto the posterior surface of the calcaneus.

Plantar aponeurosis

Medial process of tuberosity of calcaneus

Flexor digitorum brevis m.

Plantar aponeurosis

Medial process of tuberosity of calcaneus

Flexor digitorum brevis m.

Figure 5.50 Longitudinal view of the plantar aponeurosis arising from the medial process of the calcaneal tuberosity.

6

Thorax: Chest Wall and Pleura

Review of the Anatomy

Thoracic Wall

The thorax is the part of the body occupying the space between the neck and abdomen. The bony cage of the thorax is conical in shape, has a narrow apex superiorly (the superior thoracic aperture, leading to the root of the neck) and a wide base inferiorly (the inferior thoracic aperture guarded by the diaphragm). The true thoracic wall includes the thoracic cage and the intercostal muscles and the musculature of the anterolateral wall. The same structures covering its posterior aspect are considered as part of the back.

Bones of the Thoracic Wall

The bones of the thoracic wall include the sternum and the ribs. The sternum is a flat bone composed of 3 parts: the manubrium, the body, and the xiphoid process.

The manubrium superiorly has the jugular notch and, on each of its lateral sides, the clavicular notch for articulating with the clavicle. The manubrium also articulates with the first rib, the second rib, and the body of the sternum. The junction between the manubrium and the body of the sternum is also known as the sternal angle (of Louis) and is the site of the manubriosternal joint. This landmark marks the following:

- second rib articulates with the sternum
- bifurcation of the trachea
- where the aortic arch begins and ends
- the inferior border of the superior mediastinum
- the T4/ T5 vertebral level

The body of the sternum articulates with the second to seventh costal cartilages at the sternocostal joints and the xiphoid process at the xiphisternal joint.

There are 12 pair of ribs that are classified as either true or false with the last 2 termed *floating* as they do not attach to the sternum. The true ribs are the ribs 1 to 7 and directly articulate with the sternum. The false ribs are ribs 8 to 10 and are connected to the seventh rib via costal cartilages. Ribs 11 and 12 are not connected to the sternum. A typical rib consists of a head, neck, tubercle, and body. The head of the rib articulates with the superior and inferior costal facets (demifacets) of the corresponding vertebral bodies. The tubercle articulates with the transverse process of the corresponding vertebrae (except ribs 11 and 12). The body of the rib contains a costal groove along its inferior edge in which the intercostal vein, artery, and nerve are accommodated.

Intercostal Muscles

There are 3 intercostal muscles: the external intercostals, internal intercostals, and the innermost intercostals. The external intercostal muscle is located superficially, and its fiber orientation runs medially and downward in a direction in line with the external abdominal oblique muscle of the anterior abdominal wall. At the level of the sternum, the external intercostal muscle is replaced by the anterior intercostal membrane. Deep to the external intercostal muscle is the internal intercostal muscle. This muscle runs in a direction opposite the external intercostals downward and laterally, in line with the internal abdominal oblique muscle. The innermost intercostal muscle is the deepest of the intercostal muscles, running in the same direction as the internal intercostals muscle.

Intercostal Arteries, Veins, and Nerves

The intercostal arteries travel between the ribs. Each intercostal space is typically supplied by a posterior intercostal artery and a pair of anterior intercostal arteries. The anterior intercostal arteries are branches of the internal thoracic arteries, and the posterior intercostal arteries are branches of the descending thoracic aorta. In addition, the first and second intercostal spaces are usually supplied by the supreme or superior intercostal artery, which is a branch of the costocervical trunk, a branch of the subclavian artery.

The intercostal veins run alongside the intercostal arteries and nerves. Similar to the arteries, there are posterior intercostal veins that drain to the azygos/hemiazygos venous system. The anterior intercostal veins are tributaries of the internal thoracic veins. The posterior intercostal veins of the first intercostal space drain into the right and left brachiocephalic veins. The posterior intercostal veins of the second and third intercostal spaces come together and form the superior intercostal vein. The right superior intercostal vein drains into the azygos vein, and the left superior intercostal vein drains into the left brachiocephalic vein.

There are 12 pairs of thoracic spinal nerves that supply the thoracic wall. These nerves exit the intervertebral foramina and immediately divide into anterior and posterior primary rami. The anterior primary rami of T1–T11 nerves run at the intercostal spaces and are thus termed intercostal nerves. The anterior primary ramus of T12 nerve runs inferior to the 12th rib and is called the subcostal nerve. The posterior primary rami of thoracic intercostal spinal nerves run posteriorly, lateral to the articular processes of the vertebrae, and supply the joints, deep muscles of the back muscles, and their corresponding dermatomes.

The intercostal nerves give off lateral cutaneous branches in the midaxillary line and then terminate as anterior cutaneous nerves. The intercostal nerves innervate the intercostal muscles and corresponding dermatomes. In general, the intercostal veins, arteries, and nerves run between the internal and innermost intercostal muscles in the costal grooves.

Pleura

The pleura is a thin serous membrane that envelopes each lung and consists of parietal and visceral layers. The parietal pleura is subdivided into:

- costal pleura adherent to the ribs
- cervical pleura extending above the first rib into the root of the neck
- mediastinal pleura facing the mediastinum
- diaphragmatic pleura adherent to the superior surface of the diaphragm

The parietal pleura is attached to the internal surface of the thoracic wall by the endothoracic fascia. In the neck, the cervical pleura is reinforced by a condensed part of the endothoracic fascia also known as Sibson's fascia (suprapleural membrane). The visceral layer invests the lungs themselves. The costal pleura is innervated by the intercostal nerves. The mediastinal and diaphragmatic pleurae are innervated by the phrenic nerves. Thus, the parietal pleura is sensitive to pain, in contrast to the visceral pleura, which is pain insensitive but receives vasomotor innervation for stretch and respiratory reflexes via the vagus nerve.

The internal thoracic, superior phrenic, posterior intercostal, and superior intercostal arteries supply the parietal pleura, whereas the visceral pleura is supplied by the bronchial arteries.

Between the parietal and visceral pleurae is a potential space, the pleural space. The pleura is composed of mesothelial cells producing small amounts of serous fluid, which facilitate the movements of the lungs. During normal respiration, the lungs are not fully expanded and, as result, the parietal pleura is not in contact with the visceral pleura. The areas in which the parietal pleura is not in direct contact with the lung parenchyma are termed recesses, of which there are two. The costodiaphragmatic recess is formed by the reflection of costal and diaphragmatic pleurae. The costomediastinal recess is formed between the costal and mediastinal pleurae.

Technique

PECTORAL MUSCLES
RIBS
INTERCOSTAL SPACE
PLEURA
Longitudinal
  (Parasagittal)
FIG. 6.1

The patient should be supine and appropriately draped to allow for palpation of landmarks and for placing and manipulating the probe while maintaining patient privacy and comfort. Use a high-frequency linear probe (although all of the relevant anatomy can be seen using a curved array probe, resolution is much better with the linear probe and so it is better for learning the anatomy), with the marker directed toward the head.

Place the probe on the midclavicular line over the second, third or fourth intercostal space with the marker side pointing over the rib above and heel over the rib below (acoustic shadows from the ribs above and below on each side of the image).

From superficial to deep identify the following structures:

- pectoralis major
- pectoralis minor
- intercostal muscles and membranes
- hyperechoic pleural line (at the deep surface of the ribs)
- sonographic A and B lines

The pleura has a thickness of about 0.2 mm, very close to the limit of sonographic identification. However, with careful examination, both the parietal and visceral pleurae can be depicted as 2 separate echogenic lines. In general, the parietal pleura is better seen compared with the visceral pleura and appears as a fine echogenic line. With high-definition ultrasound a double line can be seen depicting the parietal pleura and endothoracic fascia. The visceral pleura,

Figure 6.1   Normal longitudinal (parasagittal) view of an intercostal space and the pleural line.

however, is more difficult to identify. It has been described as a delicate echogenic line, embedded in the near total reflection of ultrasound waves over the air-filled lung. Reflection and reverberation artifacts are the dominant imaging features of the visceral pleura and its surrounding structures. With careful observation, a back and forth shimmering movement referred to as the pleural sliding sign can be seen, in which the visceral pleura slides along the parietal pleura with respiration. The presence of pleural sliding virtually rules out pneumothorax at this location.

Occasional sonographic B lines are also seen in normal individuals. These are thin hyperechoic comet-tail reverberation artifacts perpendicular to the pleural line, which move back and forth synchronously with pleural sliding. This is probably caused by differences in acoustic impedance of alveolar air versus interstitial fluid in the alveolar walls/interalveolar septae near the lung surface. Numerous, or coalescing thickened B lines (lung rockets) indicate pulmonary edema and/or pneumonia.

Sonographic A lines are equally spaced hyperechoic lines parallel to the pleural line and are reverberation artifacts (seen with normal lungs and seen in pneumothorax).

Absence of pleural sliding indicates pneumothorax, and the location where sliding stops is referred to as the *lung point* (the edge of the pneumothorax versus normal lung/pleural space). Absence of B lines is also important in the diagnosis of pneumothorax. If any B lines are seen, even in the absence of obvious pleural sliding, the probability of pneumothorax is greatly reduced.

PECTORAL MUSCLES
RIBS
INTERCOSTAL SPACE
PLEURA
Transverse
FIG. 6.2

Starting from the probe position described above for Figure 6.1, rotate the probe 90 degrees counterclockwise so the marker points to the patient's right. Place the probe over an intercostal space with no rib shadowing as in the sagittal view and identify the following structures:

- pectoralis major
- pectoralis minor
- intercostal muscles and membranes
- hyperechoic pleural line
- sonographic A lines

Figure 6.2 Normal transverse view of an intercostal space and the pleural line.

CLINICAL APPLICATIONS

Ultrasound examination of the pleura, pleural line, and pleural sliding sign is used to screen for pneumothorax in thoracoabdominal trauma as part of the extended focused assessment with sonography for trauma (eFAST) examination.

The same techniques are also used in bedside examination for nontraumatic pneumothorax, pulmonary edema, pleural effusion, hemothorax, and hematomas. Ultrasound examination of the thorax can also detect rib fractures with fairly high accuracy, similarly bone metastasis and peripheral lung cancer infiltrating the chest wall.

7

Heart

Review of the Anatomy

Pericardium

The pericardium is a fibroserous sac that encloses the entire heart and a portion of the great vessels and is composed of 2 layers, one fibrous and one serous. The fibrous pericardium is tough and dense, forming the outermost layer of the pericardial sac. The fibrous pericardium is attached to the deep surface of the sternum by the sternopericardial ligaments (composed of condensations of mediastinal areolar tissue), to the diaphragm (inferiorly), and to the adventitial layer of the aorta and pulmonary trunk.

The serous pericardium is composed of 2 layers of mesothelial cells, the visceral and the parietal. The parietal layer of serous pericardium line the interior surface of the fibrous pericardium. The visceral pericardium is most frequently referred to as the epicardium, which forms the outermost layer of the heart. The space between the visceral and the parietal serous pericardium is the pericardial cavity. The mesothelial lining of the serous pericardium secretes pericardial fluid. The function of the pericardial fluid is to allow the heart to move more efficiently by reducing energy lost to friction.

The Heart

The heart is located within the pericardial sac. It weighs about 250 g in women and 300 g in men. The transverse diameter varies with inspiration and expiration but normally measures 8 to 9 cm in transverse diameter on a radiograph at end-maximum inspiration in the standing position. Typically, the width of the normal heart is less than one-half width of the chest. The cardiac wall possesses 3 distinct layers, the endocardium, myocardium, and epicardium. The endocardium is composed of endothelial cells and forms the inner surface of the heart that comes into contact with the blood. The myocardium is composed of myocardial cells, which contract to expel blood. The epicardium is the visceral pericardium forming the outermost layer of the heart.

Cardiac Borders

The borders of the heart are important clinically because they are used as landmarks to diagnose pathologies of the heart. The right border of the heart demarcates the inferior vena cava, right atrium, and superior vena cava. The left border of the heart delineates the left ventricle and the pulmonary trunk. The left, or pulmonary, surface is composed mainly of the left ventricle. The inferior border demarcates the right ventricle. The right ventricle forms the sternocostal surface and part of the diaphragmatic surface of the heart. The apex of the heart is located in a healthy heart at the fifth intercostal space, i.e., the point of maximal impulse of cardiac inspection/auscultation. The base of the heart is demarcated by the left atrium and a small portion of the right atrium.

Right Atrium

The right atrium has the thinnest wall of the 4 chambers of the heart. The right atrium is typically divided into 2 parts, the sinus venarum and the right atrium proper. The sinus venarum is the smooth-walled region of the right atrium, which contains the superior vena cava, the inferior vena cava, and the opening of the coronary sinus. The sinus venarum develops embryologically from the sinus venosus. The right atrium proper contains the crista terminalis, pectinate muscles, right auricular appendage, and interatrial septum.

The external surface of the right atrium is broad, triangular, and pyramidal in shape. On the right atrium there are 2 large orifices for the superior and inferior vena cavae. The superior vena cava is formed by the junction of the left and right brachiocephalic veins in the superior mediastinum. The inferior vena cava contains a small crescentic valve, the Eustachian valve. Rarely, this valve can be present as a fenestrated structure connected to the atrial vestibule (Chiari's network). In some cases, a large fenestrated valve of the inferior vena cava can be misdiagnosed as a **thrombus** (blood clot).

The anterior cardiac vein also has an opening into the right atrium. The sulcus terminalis is a shallow groove in the roof of the right atrium, which extends between the right side of the orifice of the superior vena cava and that of the inferior vena cava. The sulcus terminalis externally corresponds to a muscular ridge, the crista terminalis, internally. The crista terminalis marks the line of junction of the right atrium with the right auricle. The auricles are appendages of the atria. The sulcus terminalis contains the artery to the sinoatrial node. The pectinate muscles are slender bands of muscle that arise from the crista terminalis and fan out through the wall of the right auricle. The roof of the atrium is smooth, in contrast with that of the auricle. The right auricular appendage contains small condensed pectinate muscles, which may potentially trap a venous thrombus and, if dislodged, result in a pulmonary embolism. The interatrial septum forms the medial wall of the right atrium. Within the septum is a depressed region, the fossa ovalis, bordered by a thicker rim of muscle, the limbus fossa ovalis. The fossa ovalis marks the line of fusion between the original embryonic septum secundum and the septum primum, closing the ostium secundum in the morphologic formation of the septum. In almost 20% of individuals, the area of fusion in the interatrial septum is incomplete and an oblique fissure of communication between the 2 atria is retained. This condition is known as *probe patency* of the foramen ovale and is usually of no physiologic significance. Finally, the right atrium opens into the right ventricles via the right atrioventricular (AV) valve (tricuspid valve).

Left Atrium

The left atrium is the most posteriorly located structure of the heart. It has thicker walls than the right atrium, and its endocardium is thicker than that of the right atrium because of higher pressures. The interior of the left atrium is smooth and possesses very few pectinate muscles, which are confined to the auricle. The left auricle is relatively long and thin, resembling a pointing finger. The left atrium receives 4 or 5 pulmonary veins, 2 from the left lung and 3 from the right lung. Several venae cordis minimae are also present within the walls of the left atrium. The left atrium receives oxygenated blood from the lungs and communicates with the left ventricle via the left AV valve (mitral).

Right Ventricle

The right ventricle is the most anterior of all the heart chambers and is almost in contact with the sternum. The right ventricle has thin walls and is separated into 2 parts, the inflow and outflow parts. The inflow portion contains the tricuspid valve, papillary muscles, interventricular septum, and trabeculae carneae. The tricuspid valve possesses 3 leaflets, the anterior, posterior, and septal. The separation of the 3 leaflets may not be well delineated. The leaflets are anchored to papillary muscles within the ventricle by slender, tough chordae tendineae. The chordae tendineae are connected to a large anterior papillary muscle, a small posterior papillary muscle, and septal papillary muscles. There may be several small septal papillary muscles arising from the interventricular septum, with short chordae tendineae passing to the septal leaflet of the valve. It is important to realize that the papillary muscles and their chordae tendineae do not open the tricuspid valve; in fact, the valve opens passively because of pressure differences between the right atrium and right ventricle when the right ventricle is relaxing (diastole). The papillary muscles and chordae tendineae keep the valve leaflets (and blood within the right ventricle) from being forced or "blown" upward into the right atrium when the right ventricle contacts (systole). Blood within the right ventricle is then expelled unidirectionally through the valve of the pulmonary artery.

The right ventricle contains thick, irregular-shaped bundles of muscle the trabeculae carneae. One such bundle of muscle, the moderator band (or septomarginal trabeculation), is very prominent. This band of muscle passes from the muscular interventricular septum to the base of the anterior papillary muscle. The crista supraventricularis separates the inflow from the outflow portions of the heart. The pulmonary semilunar valve has 3 semilunar-shaped leaflets (right, left, and anterior) that join one another at the commissures. Each leaflet is strengthened at the periphery by a rim of connective tissue known as the lunule and a thickened central portion of each leaflet called the nodule. The pulmonary trunk begins at the level of the pulmonary valve and after 3 to 5 cm bifurcates into the right and left pulmonary arteries. The conus or infundibulum is the horizontal mass of muscular tissue on which two-thirds of the pulmonary valve rests.

Left Ventricle

The wall of the left ventricle is approximately 3 times thicker than the wall of the right ventricle because of its need to propel blood to the systemic circulation. Traditionally, the left ventricle has been divided into the aortic vestibule and the ventricle proper. The aortic vestibule contains the smooth portion of the interventricular septum, the membranous septum, the aortic semilunar valve, and the aortic root. The aortic semilunar valves possess 3 semilunar leaflets, right (right coronary leaflet), left (left coronary leaflet), and posterior (noncoronary leaflet). They also possess a lunule and nodule for each leaflet similar to the pulmonary valve. The ostia of the coronary arteries arise from depressions in the wall of the aorta, the aortic sinuses of Valsalva.

The left AV valve (mitral valve) rests between the left atrium and left ventricle. This valve is often called the bicuspid valve, although one may be able to distinguish an anterior leaflet, a posterior leaflet, and 2 smaller leaflets at the left and right ends of the valve orifice. However, the mitral valve typically has 2 leaflets, an anterior and a posterior, attaching via chordae tendineae to 2 papillary muscles, the posteromedial and the anterolateral. The chordae tendineae and papillary muscles keep the valve leaflets from being forced up into the atria during systole. Within the left ventricle there are muscular ridges, the trabeculae carneae.

Cardiac Valves and Their Location

The position of the cardiac valves is as follows: The pulmonary semilunar valves are typically located at the medial end of the left third costal cartilage. The aortic semilunar valve is located deep to the sternum at the level of the third intercostal space. The tricuspid valve lies behind the sternum to the right at the fourth intercostal space. The mitral valve is located deep to the sternum to the left at the fourth intercostal space.

Coronary Arteries

Right Coronary Artery

The right coronary artery arises from the anterior (right) aortic sinus of Valsalva. The artery passes between the pulmonary trunk and the edge of the right auricle and descends in the right coronary sulcus.

The first branch of the right coronary artery is the artery of the sinus node, which arises in approximately 60% of humans from the proximal portion of the right coronary artery, passing then up the medial wall of the right atrium to the junction of the superior vena cava and the right auricle, where it enters the sinus node. This artery, however, may arise from the proximal left coronary artery or be doubly supplied from both coronary arteries.

The second branch of the right coronary artery is the artery of the conus. The conus artery arises from the right coronary artery and passes to the left, around the right ventricle, at the level of the pulmonary semilunar valve. Close to the diaphragmatic surface of the heart, the right coronary artery typically gives off the right marginal artery, which supplies the inferior border of the right ventricle. The right coronary artery continues posteriorly in the AV groove and, in most cases, will descend and terminate in the posterior interventricular groove as the posterior interventricular (descending) artery. This artery supplies the inferior one-third of the interventricular septum and a portion of the inferior wall of the left ventricle. In 80% of humans, the artery of the AV node arises from the right coronary near the posterior interventricular groove.

Left Coronary Artery

The left coronary artery is a short artery arising from the posterior (left) aortic sinus of Valsalva and runs between the pulmonary trunk and ascending aorta before bifurcating into the anterior interventricular and circumflex arteries. The anterior interventricular artery is often referred to clinically in abbreviated form as the left anterior descending (LAD) artery. This vessel gives off, typically, 2 or more large diagonal branches to the anterior surface of the left ventricle. Deeply penetrating septal branches arise from the deep surface of the anterior interventricular artery and enter the muscular interventricular septum, supplying the anterior two-thirds of the septum. The posterior one-third of the septum is supplied by similar branches from the posterior descending coronary artery. The circumflex coronary artery runs in the left AV groove toward the left border and around to the base of the heart. This vessel typically gives off the left marginal artery crossing the left border of the heart supplying the left ventricular free wall.

Cardiac Veins

The coronary sinus is a small confluence of veins approximately 2 cm long, which lies at the AV groove externally and between the opening of the inferior vena cava and the tricuspid valve internally to eventually empty into the right atrium. It receives the great cardiac vein, the middle cardiac vein, and occasionally the small cardiac vein and the oblique vein of the left atrium. The opening of the coronary sinus is guarded by the valve of the coronary sinus, the Thebesian valve.

The great cardiac vein lies in the anterior interventricular groove, accompanies the left anterior interventricular artery, and drains the anterior portion of the interventricular septum and the anterior aspect of both ventricles. The middle cardiac vein lies in the posterior interventricular groove, accompanies the posterior interventricular artery, and drains the posterior part of the interventricular septum and the posterior aspect of both ventricles. The small cardiac vein lies in the AV groove next to the opening of the coronary sinus. It usually joins the right marginal vein or separately opens to the right atrium. It drains the marginal portion of the right ventricle and accompanies the right marginal artery. Not all of venous drainage of the myocardium passes into the coronary sinus. The anterior cardiac veins drain directly into the right atrium. Other venous channels within the myocardium also empty directly into the chambers of the heart by small openings in the walls, especially within the right atrium; these are called Thebesian veins or venae cordis minimae.

Conduction Tissue of the Heart

Specialized cardiac muscle fibers compose the conduction tissue of the heart that sends electrical signals to the cardiac musculature, resulting in its contraction. The major specialized cardiac conduction muscle fibers are the sinoatrial and AV nodes, as well as the bundles of His and Purkinje fibers.

The sinoatrial node is located at the junction of the base of the superior vena cava with the right auricle. The AV node is situated deep to the musculature of the medial wall of the right atrium adjacent to the septal leaflet of the tricuspid valve. The bundle of His (common AV bundle) exits inferiorly from the AV node through the central fibrous body, curving inferior to the membranous septum to reach the superior margin of the muscular interventricular septum. The bundle of His passes for a short distance on the superior aspect of the interventricular septum and then divides into a broad left branch to the left ventricle and a narrow right branch, which passes into the right ventricle. A subendocardial network of specialized cardiac muscle cells (Purkinje fibers) arises from the left and right bundle branches. This network conveys the excitatory impulse from the branches of the common bundle (of His) to the myocardium of the ventricles.

Technique

Cardiac ultrasound (US) imaging, often referred to as **echocardiography**, has been integrated into the functional cardiac evaluation of cardiovascular disease. Although a very basic imaging modality, it provides vast amounts of information pertaining to cardiac structures and function. The 2 most common types of cardiac US imaging are transthoracic echocardiography and transesophageal echocardiography. In this chapter we will describe the different transthoracic approaches, namely, apical, parasternal long and short axis, and subxiphoid 4-chamber view.

APICAL 4-CHAMBER VIEW
FIG. 7.1

To obtain the apical view, place the patient in a supine position. In cases in which it is difficult to visualize the heart, placing the patient in a left lateral decubitus position often greatly improves the image. Place the probe face lateral to the nipple line at the point of the cardiac apex or apical pulse. The transducer should be tilted 60 degrees toward the right shoulder, and the probe indicator should be pointed toward the patient's

left axilla. Identify the interventricular septum separating the right and left ventricles. Identify the mitral and tricuspid valves. The tricuspid valve is located more inferior than the mitral valve in the horizontal plane, giving the impression that the left ventricle is longer that the right ventricle. In addition, the ventricles appear to sit on top of the atria. This is because the transducer is closer to the ventricles than the atria at this location.

PARASTERNAL LONG AXIS VIEW
FIG. 7.2

To obtain the parasternal long axis view, place the probe face just to the left of the sternum in the third, fourth, or fifth intercostal space (most commonly fourth). The nonmarker side of the probe should be pointed toward the patient's right shoulder when the screen marker is on the left of the display image (so that the marker side of the probe is directed toward the 4-o'clock position). When the screen marker is on the right side of the display, the marker side of the probe should be directed toward the right shoulder. This orients the probe/US beam along the long axis of the left

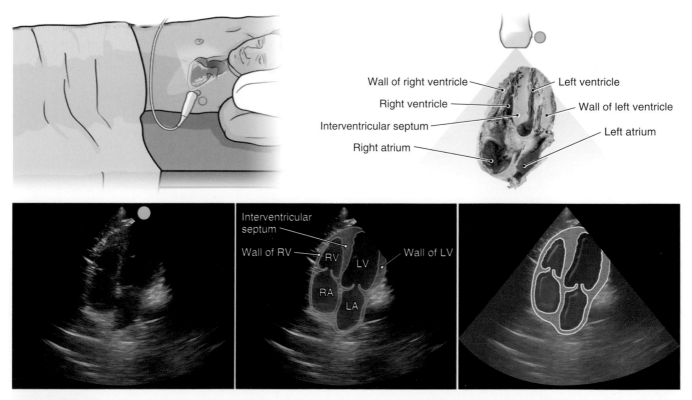

Wall of right ventricle — Left ventricle
Right ventricle — Wall of left ventricle
Interventricular septum — Left atrium
Right atrium

Interventricular septum
Wall of RV — RV — LV — Wall of LV
RA
LA

Figure 7.1 Apical 4-chamber view of the heart. LA, left atrium; LV, left ventricle; RA, right atrium; RV, right ventricle.

ventricle and displays the image as shown in Figure 7.2. Adjust probe position up or down one intercostal space at a time as needed, until an image of the heart as shown in Figure 7.2 can be best seen. In this view the right ventricle is located more superficially to the top of the image, giving the impression that the right ventricle is sitting on top of the left ventricle. The right atrium is not visible. The posterior free wall of the left ventricle and adjacent posterior pericardium should be identified in the far field. The left atrium, mitral valve, inflow tract of the left ventricle, outflow tract of the left ventricle, aortic valve, and ascending aorta should be identified. The interventricular septum and outflow tract of the right ventricle should be seen in the near field. The descending thoracic aorta can often be seen just posterior to the left atrium near the position of the mitral valve annulus. The apex of the left ventricle should be beyond the edge of the display image to the left.

PARASTERNAL SHORT AXIS VIEW FIG. 7.3

To obtain the parasternal short axis view, follow the previous instructions to get a long axis view and then rotate the probe 90 degrees clockwise. The nonmarker side of the probe should be pointed toward the patient's left shoulder when the screen marker is on the left of the display image (so that the marker side of the probe is directed toward the

8-o'clock position). When the screen marker is on the right side of the display, the marker side of the probe should be directed toward the left shoulder. This orients the probe/US beam along the short axis of the left ventricle, and the heart is seen in a plane perpendicular to the parasternal long axis as displayed in Figure 7.3. Adjust probe position up or down one intercostal space at a time as needed, until an image of the left ventricle appears in a circular pattern in the far field while the crescent-shaped right ventricle can be seen in the near field. Fan the probe superiorly toward the base of the heart to view and identify the aortic valve. In this view the 3 leaflets of the aortic valve are evident as the aortic valve opens and closes. During closure of the aortic valve the aortic leaflets come together, and this gives the characteristic appearance of the "Mercedes Benz" sign. The aortic valve possesses 3 leaflets, the right coronary leaflet, the left coronary leaflet, and the posterior noncoronary leaflet. The right coronary leaflet is the most anterior leaflet located next (beneath in the image) to the right ventricle and pulmonary valve. The noncoronary leaflet is located adjacent to the right atrium and interatrial septum and the left coronary leaflet is located in front of the left atrium. Moving the probe inferiorly toward the apex the mitral valve can be visualized with its characteristic "fish mouth" appearance inside the left ventricle. Tilting the probe further inferiorly toward the apex of the heart the 2 papillary muscles (posteromedial and anterolateral) can be visualized.

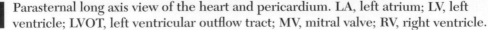

Figure 7.2 Parasternal long axis view of the heart and pericardium. LA, left atrium; LV, left ventricle; LVOT, left ventricular outflow tract; MV, mitral valve; RV, right ventricle.

SUBXIPHOID 4-CHAMBER VIEW FIG. 7.4

The subxiphoid 4-chamber view uses the liver as a sonographic window to view the heart and pericardium. If the patient can cooperate, flexing the knees to 90 degrees and placing the soles of the feet on the bed relaxes the abdominal musculature. To obtain this view, place the probe face just to the right of the midline 2 to 4 cm below the xiphoid process, depending on the width of the subcostal arch. The probe should be far enough below the xiphoid process so that the sides of the probe face are not pressing against ribs/costal cartilages. Next, exert pressure directly posteriorly, and then with a scooping motion, flatten the probe against the abdominal wall directing the US beam upward and slightly toward the left shoulder. Adjust probe position and tilt until the liver, right and left ventricles, right and left atria, and pericardium can be identified. The right ventricle appears to be on the top of the picture because it is the closest to the probe. If needed, increase the depth setting until the posterior pericardium adjacent to the free wall of the left ventricle can be clearly seen in the far field. If possible, ask the patient to take a deep breath, which brings the heart closer to the probe and improves image quality.

Note: When a microconvex phased array (cardiac) probe is used, many US units automatically place the screen marker dot to the right of the screen image rather than to the left of the screen image as in all other applications. If the screen marker dot is on the left of the image as usual, then the marker side of the probe should be directed toward the patient's right axilla to obtain display images as shown in Figure 7.1. If the marker dot is on the right of the screen image, then the marker side of the probe should be directed toward the patient's left flank to obtain the same image orientation on the display.

CLINICAL APPLICATIONS

Echocardiography is used to examine the pericardium, heart, and cardiac valves in a variety of conditions. The extended focused assessment with sonography for trauma (eFAST) examination is used in the setting of blunt and/or penetrating trauma of the thorax and abdomen. The subxiphoid 4-chamber view or the parasternal long axis view are commonly used in the eFAST examination to determine if there is free fluid accumulating in the pericardial space (hemopericardium or pericardial effusion). The **eFAST examination** and potential findings are discussed in detail in Chapter 12.

Cardiac tamponade is the compression of the heart that occurs when the pericardial sac, which resists sudden distention, contains excessive fluid or blood. When an excess of fluid is present, the heart cannot fill properly in diastole; therefore, cardiac output is compromised. In addition to observing fluid accumulation in the pericardial space, diastolic collapse of the right ventricle can be observed with ultrasound in the setting of cardiac tamponade.

The contraction of the ventricles can be observed in real time with US, allowing for detection of global or focal wall motion abnormalities such as those produced by coronary artery disease or ventricular failure. Doppler technologies are used to observe regurgitant flow across incompetent valves and to measure systolic flow velocity across stenotic valves. **Pericardiocentesis** is the removal of fluid from the pericardial sac so as to relieve the problem of tamponade. Although pericardiocentesis can be performed using landmarks alone, US-guided pericardiocentesis allows for visualization of the effusion, as well as the needle path and guidewire during the procedure, and has been shown to reduce clinical errors such as pneumothorax. US can also be used to detect the presence of atrial mural thrombi and cardiac tumors such as left atrial myxomas.

Figure 7.3   Parasternal short axis view of the heart at the level of the aortic valve. LCL, left coronary leaflet; NCL, noncoronary leaflet; RCL, right coronary leaflet.

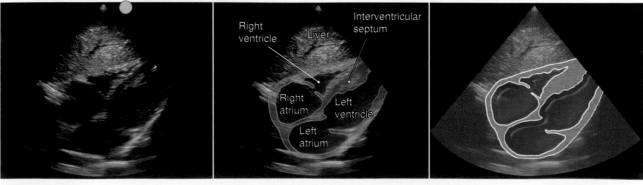

Figure 7.4   Subxiphoid 4-chamber view of the heart and pericardium.

8

Abdomen

Abdominal Wall

Review of the Anatomy

Anterior Abdominal Wall

The abdominal wall is separated topographically into 9 divisions by 2 longitudinal and 2 transverse planes. These are right hypochondriac, epigastric, left hypochondriac, right lumbar, umbilical, left lumbar, right inguinal (iliac), hypogastric (pubic), and left inguinal (iliac). In addition, the abdominal wall can also be segregated into right and left upper quadrants and right and left lower quadrants via vertical and horizontal planes that form 4 quadrants. The abdominal wall is composed of skin, subcutaneous tissue, fat, muscles and their **aponeuroses** and deep fascia, extraperitoneal fat, and parietal peritoneum.

Fasciae, Ligaments, and Muscles

The fascia of the anterior abdominal wall is composed of superficial and deep layers. The superficial layer contains a superficial fatty layer (Camper's fascia) and a deep membranous layer (Scarpa's fascia). **Camper's fascia** lies over the inguinal ligament and merges with the superficial fascia of the thigh. It continues over the pubis and perineum as the superficial layer of the superficial perineal fascia. **Scarpa's fascia** joins with the membranous layer, **Colle's fascia**, inferiorly, and medially with the superficial fascia of the penis and over the scrotum (tunica dartos). The deep fascia continues over the spermatic cord at the superficial inguinal ring by conjoining with the external spermatic fascia. The deep fascia also connects with the deep fascia of the penis, known as **Buck fascia**, located over the penis, and extends over the pubis and perineum as the deep perineal fascia.

In the anterolateral abdominal wall there is the presence of 5 bilaterally paired muscles. Of these muscles, 3 are flat muscles, including the external abdominal oblique, internal abdominal oblique, and transversus abdominis. Two muscle groups are vertically oriented, the rectus abdominis and pyramidalis. The muscle fibers of the 3 flat muscles are oriented in a diagonal and perpendicular fashion to each other. These 3 flat muscles extend anteriorly and medially as a well-fortified sheetlike aponeuroses. The fusion of the aponeurosis of the external abdominal oblique, internal abdominal oblique, and transversus abdominis muscles forms a midline avascular connective tissue white line known as the **linea alba**. The linea alba is positioned between the 2 rectus abdominis muscles and stretches from the xiphoid process to the pubic symphysis. A curved line along the lateral border of the rectus abdominis is called the linea semilunaris. A crescent-shaped line called the linea semicircularis or arcuate line forms the lower border of the posterior layer of the rectus sheath located inferior to the level of the iliac crest. The fusion of the aponeuroses of the external abdominal oblique, internal abdominal oblique, and transversus abdominis muscles form the **rectus sheath**. It surrounds the rectus abdominis and occasionally the pyramidalis muscle. It also contains the superior and inferior epigastric vessels and the ventral primary rami of thoracic nerves 7 to 12. Superior to the arcuate line, the anterior layer of the rectus sheath is formed by the aponeuroses of the external and internal abdominal oblique muscles and by the aponeuroses of the external, internal abdominal oblique, and transversus abdominis muscles inferior to the arcuate line. The posterior layer of the rectus sheath is formed by the aponeuroses of the internal abdominal oblique and the transverse muscles above the arcuate line. The rectus abdominis connects to transversalis fascia below the arcuate line.

Inguinal Region

The inguinal (Hesselbach's) triangle is bounded medially by the linea semilunaris, laterally by the inferior epigastric vessels, and inferiorly by the inguinal ligament. The superficial inguinal ring is a triangular opening in the aponeurosis of the external abdominal oblique muscle located lateral to the pubic tubercle. On the other hand, the deep inguinal ring is found in the transversalis fascia, located lateral to the inferior epigastric vessels. The **inguinal canal** starts at the deep inguinal ring and continues to the superficial ring where it terminates. This canal carries the spermatic cord or the round ligament of the uterus and the genital branch of the genitofemoral nerve. Both of these structures travel through the deep inguinal ring and the inguinal canal. Although the ilioinguinal nerve is carried through a portion of the inguinal canal and the superficial inguinal ring, it does not travel through the deep inguinal ring. The anterior wall of the inguinal canal is created by the aponeuroses of the external and internal abdominal oblique muscles. The posterior wall is formed by the aponeurosis of the transversus abdominis muscle and transversalis fascia.

The superior surface (roof) is formed by arching fibers of the internal abdominal oblique and transversus abdominis muscles. The inferior surface (floor) is formed by the inguinal and lacunar ligaments.

Nerves

The anterior and anterolateral abdominal wall is innervated by the anterior divisions of the 7th to 11th intercostal nerves, known as thoracoabdominal nerves. In addition, the inferior segment of the anterolateral wall is supplied by additional nerves including the subcostal, iliohypogastric, and ilioinguinal nerves. The subcostal nerve is the ventral ramus of the 12th thoracic nerve that supplies innervation to the muscles of the anterior abdominal wall. The iliohypogastric nerve emerges from the first lumbar nerve and innervates the internal oblique and transverse muscles of the abdomen. It subsequently branches into a lateral cutaneous branch to supply the skin of the lateral side of the buttocks and hips and an anterior cutaneous branch to supply the skin superior to the pubic symphysis. The ilioinguinal nerve arises from the first lumbar nerve and pierces the internal oblique muscle near the deep inguinal ring. It travels alongside the spermatic cord through the inguinal canal and superficial inguinal ring to provide innervation to the internal abdominal oblique and transversus abdominis muscles. In addition, the ilioinguinal nerve contributes to giving off the femoral branch, which innervates the upper and medial parts of the anterior thigh, and the anterior scrotal nerve, which innervates the skin of the root of the penis (or the skin of the mons pubis) and the anterior portion of the scrotum (or the labium majus).

Vasculature

The superior epigastric artery emerges from the internal thoracic artery, enters the rectus sheath, and courses inferiorly on the posterior border of the rectus abdominis to eventually join with the inferior epigastric artery within the rectus abdominis. The inferior epigastric artery emerges from the external iliac artery superior to the inguinal ligament and enters the rectus sheath to ascend between the rectus abdominis and the posterior layer of the rectus sheath. The inferior epigastric artery subsequently joins with the superior epigastric artery and supplies collateral circulation between the subclavian and external iliac arteries. It also branches into the cremasteric artery, which travels alongside the spermatic cord. The superficial epigastric artery branches from the femoral artery and courses superiorly toward the umbilicus over the inguinal ligament to become continuous with branches of the inferior epigastric artery. The thoracoepigastric veins are longitudinal venous connections between the lateral thoracic vein and the superficial epigastric vein.

Lymphatic Drainage

Lymphatics in the area superior to the umbilicus empty into the axillary lymph nodes. The lymphatics in the area below the umbilicus empty into the superficial inguinal nodes. The superficial inguinal lymph nodes obtain lymph from the lower abdominal wall, buttocks, penis, scrotum, labium majus, and the lower parts of the vagina and anal canal. Their efferent vessels predominately gain access to the external iliac nodes and, ultimately, the lumbar (aortic) nodes.

Technique

Rectus Abdominis and Rectus Sheath

RECTUS ABDOMINIS
RECTUS SHEATH
Transverse
FIG. 8.1

With the patient in the supine position and properly draped, place the probe centered at the midline, midway between xiphoid and umbilicus. Identify the skin, superficial fascia, hyperechoic anterior layer of rectus abdominis, medial halves of right and left rectus abdominis muscles, posterior layer of rectus sheath, and transversalis fascia. Identify the centered echogenic linea alba between the medial edges of right and left rectus abdominis muscles. Trace the thin layer of hypoechoic extraperitoneal fat between transversalis fascia and parietal peritoneum.

External Abdominal Oblique, Internal Abdominal Oblique, and Transversus Abdominus

EXTERNAL ABDOMINAL OBLIQUE
INTERNAL ABDOMINAL OBLIQUE
TRANSVERSUS ABDOMINIS
Transverse
FIG. 8.2

With the patient in the supine position and properly draped, place the probe about midway between the xiphoid process and umbilicus, just lateral to the lateral edge of rectus abdominis muscle at the linea semilunaris. Slide the probe medially until the rectus abdominis is identified,

Figure 8.1 Normal transverse view, about midway between the xiphoid process and the umbilicus, of the rectus abdominis muscles, rectus sheath, linea alba, transversalis fascia, extraperitoneal fat, and parietal peritoneum.

then slide back laterally until the rectus muscle disappears just off the screen image. Adjust the probe and tilt and angle until the 3 layers of abdominal wall muscles are clearly visible. Adjust the probe as necessary and angle to visualize the hyperechoic transversalis fascia and parietal peritoneum at the deep surface of transversus abdominis muscle. Note the hyperechoic reflection and shadowing from gas in the gastrointestinal track deep to the parietal peritoneum.

Figure 8.2 Normal transverse view, midway between the xiphoid process and umbilicus, of the external abdominal oblique, transversus abdominis, transversalis fascia, and parietal peritoneum.

CLINICAL APPLICATIONS

Hernias

Epigastric hernia is a type of hernia situated at the anterolateral abdominal wall in which extraperitoneal fat or portion of the greater omentum or portion of the small intestines protrude through a defect in the linea alba superior to the umbilicus. Complications of such herniation include strangulation or incarceration of the small intestines.

Spigelian hernia (lateral ventral hernia) is a type of hernia of the anterolateral abdominal wall situated at the semilunar line. The diagnosis of a Spigelian hernia is confirmed with ultrasound (US) or computed tomography scan. The clinical presentation is dependent on the composition of the hernial sac and the degree and type of herniation. The most common presenting symptom is pain.

Incisional hernia is another hernia subtype of the anterolateral abdominal wall where the abdominal viscera extends out of a defect in the abdominal wall resulting from surgery or trauma. These types of hernias commonly occur after open abdominal operations in about 5% to 15% of patients. It has also been found that the incidence of very large or giant hernias increases with increases in the obesity of the population and the complexity of abdominal surgeries.

Transversus Abdominis Plane Block

Transversus abdominis plane block (TAPB) is a US-guided block that is used to block typically T9 to T10 nerves. TAPB with US guidance is used to accurately guide the needle bevel into a plane between internal abdominal oblique and transversus abdominis muscles to provide local anesthetic for abdominal wall incisions medial to the block. This block is indicated for several surgical procedures such as hernia repair, open appendectomy, caesarian section, total abdominal hysterectomy, and radical prostatectomy.

Peritoneum, Gastrointestinal Tract, and Liver

Review of the Anatomy

Peritoneum and Peritoneal Cavity

The peritoneum is formed by a serous membrane, which consists of mesothelial cells. It has 2 parts, the parietal and the visceral peritoneum. The parietal peritoneum lies over the abdominal and pelvic walls and the inferior aspect of the diaphragm, whereas the visceral peritoneum drapes over the abdominal viscera.

The parietal and visceral layers of the peritoneum form a potential space enabling the free movement of the abdominal viscera. The peritoneal cavity in males is a closed cavity; however, in females the peritoneal cavity is open through the vagina, uterine tubes, and uterus where it contains a small amount of peritoneal fluid. The peritoneum is innervated by the phrenic, lower intercostal, subcostal, iliohypogastric, and ilioinguinal nerves, which causes it to be sensitive to pain, in contrast to visceral peritoneum, which is insensitive to pain.

The parietal and visceral peritoneum create peritoneal reflections across the abdominal viscera. These reflections are the lesser and greater omenta, mesentery proper, transverse and sigmoid mesocolon, and the mesoappendix.

The **lesser omentum** is a dual layer of peritoneum from the porta hepatis of the liver and continues to the lesser curvature of the stomach and the beginning of the duodenum. The hepatogastric and hepatoduodenal ligaments compose the lesser omentum. They also form the anterior wall of the lesser sac of the peritoneal cavity and transmit the left and right gastric vessels, which course within the 2 layers along the lesser curvature. The lesser omentum has a free right margin that accommodates the proper hepatic artery, bile duct, and portal vein.

The **greater omentum** suspends down from the greater curvature of the stomach, draping over the transverse colon and other abdominal viscera. It transmits the right and left gastroepiploic vessels along the greater curvature of the stomach and seals the neck of a hernial sac, preventing the coils of the small intestine from entering the space. The greater omentum attaches to regions of inflammation and encases itself around inflamed organs, thus preventing serious diffuse peritonitis.

The greater omentum is often defined to encompass the following peritoneal ligaments: gastrosplenic, gastrophrenic, and gastrocolic. The splenorenal ligament is also considered by some authors as part of the greater omentum. The gastrosplenic ligament stretches from the left portion of the greater curvature of the stomach to the hilus of the spleen and contains the short gastric and left gastroepiploic vessels. The gastrophrenic ligament travels from the upper surface of the greater curvature of the stomach to the diaphragm. The gastrocolic ligament runs from the greater curvature of the stomach to the transverse colon. Finally, the splenorenal ligament travels from the hilum of the spleen to the left kidney and holds the splenic vessels and the tail of the pancreas.

The mesentery of the small intestine or mesentery proper is a doublefold of peritoneum that supports the jejunum and the ileum from the posterior abdominal wall and carries nerves, blood vessels, and lymphatics to and from the small intestine. It forms a root that stretches from the duodenojejunal flexure to the right iliac fossa. It has a free border that surrounds the small intestine and includes the superior mesenteric and intestinal (jejunal and ileal) vessels, nerves, and lymphatics.

The transverse mesocolon adjoins the posterior surface of the transverse colon to the posterior abdominal wall. It combines with the greater omentum to form the gastrocolic ligament and encloses the middle colic vessels, nerves, and lymphatics. The sigmoid mesocolon links the sigmoid colon to the pelvic wall and encompasses the sigmoid vessels. The mesoappendix connects the appendix to the mesentery of the ileum and contains the appendicular vessels.

The phrenicocolic ligament travels from the left colic flexure to the diaphragm.

The falciform ligament is a peritoneal fold that adheres the liver to the diaphragm and the anterior abdominal wall. It also contains the round ligament of the liver and the paraumbilical vein, which adjoin the left branch of the portal vein with the subcutaneous veins at the umbilicus.

The round ligament of the liver (ligamentum teres hepatis) lies in the free margin of the falciform ligament and travels superiorly from the umbilicus to the inferior (visceral) surface of the liver, lying in the fissure that forms the left boundary of the quadrate lobe of the liver. Embryologically, it is a remnant of the left umbilical vein, which carries oxygenated blood from the placenta to the left branch of the portal vein in the fetus. (The right umbilical vein is obliterated during the embryonic period.)

The coronary ligament is a peritoneal reflection, which originates from the diaphragmatic border of the liver onto the diaphragm and encloses a triangular area of the right lobe. It has right and left extensions that create the right and left triangular ligaments.

The ligamentum venosum is an embryological remnant of the ductus venosus. It is fibrous in nature and is situated in the fissure on the inferior portion of the liver, which forms the left boundary of the caudate lobe of the liver.

The umbilical folds are 5 folds of peritoneum below the umbilicus, including the median, medial, and lateral umbilical folds. The rectouterine fold courses from the cervix of the uterus, along the side of the rectum, to the posterior pelvic wall, which creates the rectouterine pouch of Douglas. The ileocecal fold extends from the terminal ileum to the cecum.

Gastrointestinal Viscera

Stomach

The stomach is completely draped over by the peritoneum and is located in the left hypochondriac and epigastric regions. The stomach has a greater and lesser curvature, anterior and posterior walls, cardiac and pyloric openings, and cardiac and angular notches. It is divided into 4 sections: cardia, fundus, body, and pylorus.

The cardia is the part of the stomach surrounding the cardiac orifice. The *fundus* is the area of the stomach inferior to the apex of the heart at the left diaphragmatic dome, at the level of the fifth rib. The body occupies the major part of the stomach and is the area between the fundus and the pyloric antrum. The *pylorus* is further subdivided into the pyloric antrum and pyloric canal. The pyloric orifice is encompassed by the pyloric sphincter, which is a band of thickened circular smooth muscle that controls the rate of release of stomach contents into the duodenum. Constriction of the sphincter is regulated by sympathetic stimulation and relaxed by parasympathetic action. The stomach receives arterial supply from the right and left gastric, right and left gastroepiploic, and short gastric arteries. As the stomach experiences contraction, it is distinguished by the appearance of longitudinal folds of mucous membrane, known as **rugae**. The gastric canal, a grooved channel along the lesser curvature formed by the rugae, directs fluids toward the pylorus. The stomach also yields hydrochloric acid and a protein-digesting enzyme, pepsin, in its fundus and body. In addition, it synthesizes the hormone gastrin, which stimulates the release of gastric acid in the pyloric antrum via parasympathetic fibers from the vagus nerve.

Small Intestine

The small intestine extends from the pyloric aperture to the ileocecal junction. The process of complete digestion and absorption of contents of digestion and water, electrolytes, and minerals such as calcium and iron take place in the small intestine. The small intestine is divided into 3 regions: duodenum, jejunum, and ileum.

Duodenum

The duodenum is a C-shaped tube surrounding the head of the pancreas. Among the other 3 regions, the duodenum is the shortest (25 cm long or 12 fingerbreadths in length) but widest portion of the small intestine. Other than the proximal portion of the duodenum, the remainder is retroperitoneal. The proximal region is connected to the liver by the hepatoduodenal ligament of the lesser omentum. The arterial supply of the duodenum is from branches of the celiac and superior mesenteric arteries.

The duodenum is divided into 4 parts:

1. *Superior (first) part:* This portion has a mobile section, known as the duodenal cap, into which the pylorus retracts.
2. *Descending (second) part:* This contains the juncture of the foregut and midgut, where the common bile and main pancreatic ducts open. It also contains the greater papilla, where the terminal ends of the bile and main pancreatic ducts are located, and the lesser papilla, which lies 2 cm above the greater papilla and marks the opening of the accessory pancreatic duct.
3. *Transverse (third) part:* This is the longest part, and it traverses the inferior vena cava, aorta, and vertebral column to the left. It is intersected anteriorly by the superior mesenteric vessels.
4. *Ascending (fourth) part:* This part of the duodenum ascends to the left of the aorta to the level of the second lumbar vertebra and stops at the duodenojejunal junction, which is fixed in position by the suspensory ligament of Treitz, a surgical landmark. This fibromuscular band is linked to the right crus of the diaphragm.

Jejunum

The jejunum is located in the proximal two-fifths of the small intestine, whereas the ileum is situated in the distal three-fifths. The jejunum is emptier, wider, and thicker walled when compared with the ileum. The jejunum has the valvelike tall, circular, and closely packed folds called the plicae circulares. It has no **Peyer's patches**, which are collections of lymphoid tissue. The jejunum also possesses some luminous areas called windows between the blood vessels of its mesentery. When compared with the ileum, the jejunum has less conspicuous arterial arcades in its mesentery. However, it has longer vasa recta (straight arteries, or arteriae rectae).

Ileum

The ileum is longer than the jejunum and resides in the false pelvis in the right lower quadrant of the abdomen. It is distinguished by the presence of Peyer's patches in its distal portion, shorter plicae circulares and vasa recta, and more mesenteric fat and arterial arcades when compared with the jejunum. The ileocecal fold is the bloodless fold of Treves.

Large Intestine

The large intestine extends from the ileocecal junction to the anus and is nearly 1.5 m long. It is made up of the cecum, appendix, colon, rectum, and anal canal. The main role is to convert the liquid contents of the ileum into semi-solid feces by absorbing water, salts, and electrolytes. It also stores and lubricates feces with mucus.

Cecum

It is the blind pouch of the large intestine. It is located in the right iliac fossa and is often surrounded by peritoneum but without a mesentery.

Appendix

This is a narrow, hollow, muscular tube with a large collection of lymphoid tissue in its wall. The appendix hangs from the terminal ileum by a small mesentery, the mesoappendix, which encompasses the appendicular vessels. When inflamed, the appendix can be a cause of spasm and distention, leading to pain that is referred to the periumbilical region and moves down and to the right lower quadrant. The appendix has a base that is located deep to the **McBurney's point**, which occurs at the junction of the lateral one-third of the line between the right anterior superior iliac spine and the umbilicus.

Rectum and Anal Canal

These extend from the juncture of the sigmoid colon to the anus. They are described as pelvic organs.

Colon

The colon has ascending and descending portions that are retroperitoneal and transverse and a sigmoid portion that is surrounded by peritoneum. The superior mesenteric artery and vagus nerve supply the ascending and transverse parts of the colon, whereas the descending and sigmoid parts of the colon are supplied by the inferior mesenteric artery and the pelvic splanchnic nerves. The colon is characterized by the following:

- *Teniae coli:* These are 3 narrow bands of the outer longitudinal muscular coat.
- *Sacculations or haustra:* These are produced by the teniae, which are slightly shorter than the gut.
- *Epiploic appendages:* These are peritoneum-covered sacs of fat, connected in rows along the teniae.

Liver

The liver is the largest visceral organ and the largest gland in the human body. It plays an important role in the synthesis and secretion of bile to emulsify fats; detoxification (by filtering the blood to remove bacteria and foreign particles that have crossed the intestinal mucosa); storage of carbohydrate as glycogen (to later break down to glucose); synthesis and sequestration of lipids as triglycerides; plasma protein synthesis (albumin and globulin); production of blood coagulants (fibrinogen and prothrombin), anticoagulants (heparin), and bile pigments (bilirubin and biliverdin) from the breakdown of hemoglobin; storage for blood and platelets; and storage of certain vitamins, iron, and copper. In the fetus, the liver plays a pivotal role in the synthesis of red blood cells.

The liver is enclosed by peritoneum and is joined to the diaphragm by the coronary and falciform ligaments and the right and left triangular ligaments. It has an exposed area on the diaphragmatic surface, which is limited by layers of the coronary ligament but without peritoneum. The liver has a dual blood supply receiving oxygenated blood from the hepatic artery and deoxygenated, nutrient-rich, sometimes toxin-containing, blood from the portal vein. It also contains a group of vessels grouped together: the hepatic artery, branch of the portal vein, and bile duct, together commonly known as the **portal triad**. The liver is enclosed by a connective tissue sheath called the perivascular fibrous capsule. The liver is divided, based on hepatic drainage and blood supply, into the right and left lobes by the fossae for the gallbladder and the inferior vena cava. (These lobes correspond to the functional units or hepatic segments.)

Lobes of the Liver

The lobes of the liver include:

- *Right lobe*: It is divided into anterior and posterior segments, each of which is further subdivided into superior and inferior areas or segments.

*   *Left lobe*: It is divided into medial and lateral segments, each of which is subdivided into superior and inferior areas (segments). It consists of the medial superior (caudate lobe), medial inferior (quadrate lobe), lateral superior, and lateral inferior segments. The quadrate lobe receives oxygenated blood from the left hepatic artery and drains bile into the left hepatic duct, whereas the caudate lobe receives oxygenated blood from the right and left hepatic arteries and drains bile into both right and left hepatic ducts.

Fissures and Ligaments of the Liver

These include an H-shaped group of fissures:

*   *Fissure for the round ligament* (ligamentum teres hepatis), located between the lateral aspect of the left lobe and the quadrate lobe.

*   *Fissure for the ligamentum venosum*, located between the lateral aspect of the left lobe and the caudate lobe.
*   *Fossa for the gallbladder*, located between the quadrate lobe and the major part of the right lobe.
*   *Fissure for the inferior vena cava*, located between the caudate lobe and the major part of the right lobe.
*   *Porta hepatis*. This transverse fissure is situated on the visceral surface of the liver between the quadrate and caudate lobes and contains the hepatic ducts, hepatic arteries, branches of the portal vein, hepatic nerves, and lymphatic vessels.

Technique

**LEFT LOBE OF LIVER
LEFT PORTAL VEIN
INFERIOR VENA CAVA
EPIGASTRIC**
Transverse
FIG. 8.3

With the patient in the supine position and properly draped, place the probe transversely to the right of the midline of epigastrium with the beam aimed slightly up. The liver will appear with a speckled pattern and a hyperechoic halo (sometimes called "train-tracks" when portal branches are seen in their long axis) around the portal veins (periportal connective tissue/fat). Identify the caudate lobe separating the inferior vena cava and left portal vein (and ascending branch of left portal vein). There is a hyperechoic line in the fissure between caudate and left liver lobe demarcating the ligamentum venosum (the patient should be asked to take a deep breath and hold while you are scanning the liver).

**INFERIOR VENA CAVA
HEPATIC VEINS
SUBCOSTAL**
Transverse
FIG. 8.4

With the patient in the supine position, place the probe transversely under the right costal margin with the beam aimed up, following the inferior vena cava and adjusting the tilt and angle when hepatic veins are identified. To differentiate between hepatic and portal veins, notice that there is no halo or train tracks around hepatic veins entering the inferior vena cava. Attempt to identify the left, middle, and right hepatic veins.

Figure 8.3   Epigastric transverse view of the left liver lobe, left portal vein and branches, caudate lobe, inferior vena cava, and ligamentum venosum.

171

LEFT LIVER LOBE
CAUDATE LOBE
PORTAL VEIN
COMMON HEPATIC
   ARTERY
SUBCOSTAL
Longitudinal
   (Parasagittal)
FIG. 8.5

With the patient in the supine position, place the probe in longitudinal orientation to right of midline under the costal margin. Adjust the probe and tilt/position it to identify the left lobe of the liver and caudate lobe. Identify the portal vein emerging from behind the neck of the pancreas as a continuation of the superior mesenteric vein below, accompanied by the common hepatic artery.

PORTAL TRIAD
INFERIOR VENA CAVA
AORTA
SUBCOSTAL
Transverse
   (Oblique)
FIG. 8.6

With the patient in the supine position, place the probe slightly oblique to the transverse plane of the abdomen and parallel to the right side of the costal margin (marker should be pointing to the right, although some clinical protocols have the marker pointing to the left shoulder). Identify and follow the portal vein to the porta hepatis and adjust and tilt/angle to see the "Mickey Mouse" sign. This sign refers to the head being the portal vein, right ear is the bile duct, and the left ear is the proper hepatic artery. The inferior vena cava should be seen posterior to the portal vein (omental foramen) and the aorta just to the left of the body of the lumbar vertebra.

PORTAL VEIN
INFERIOR VENA CAVA
SUBCOSTAL
Longitudinal
   (Oblique)
FIG. 8.7

With the patient in the supine position, place the probe under the right side of the costal margin oriented along the longitudinal axis of the body. Rotate the probe counterclockwise to oblique longitudinal orientation (the portal vein crosses obliquely from left to right) to lie along the long axis of the portal vein. Tilt up/down and left/right to identify the portal vein approaching and entering the liver. The inferior vena cava posteriorly has a vertical course, so it is not parallel to the portal vein for more than a few centimeters.

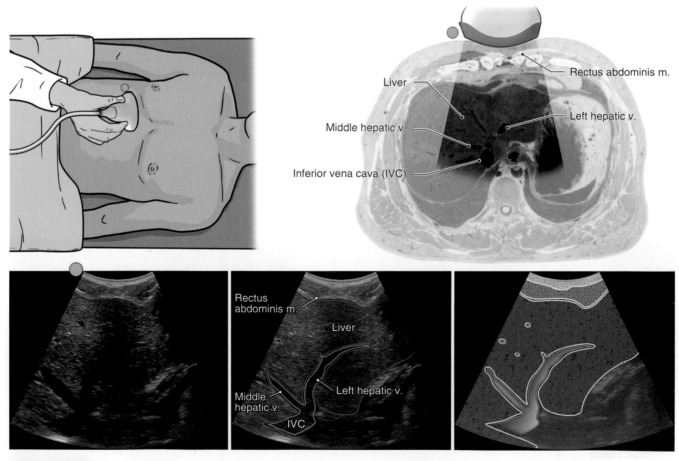

Rectus abdominis m.

Liver

Left hepatic v.

Middle hepatic v.

Inferior vena cava (IVC)

Rectus abdominis m.

Liver

Middle hepatic v.

Left hepatic v.

IVC

 Figure 8.4 Subcostal transverse view of the inferior vena cava receiving the middle and left hepatic veins.

DIVISION OF PORTAL VEIN
RIGHT AND LEFT PORTAL VEINS
INFERIOR VENA CAVA
SUBCOSTAL
Transverse
FIG. 8.8

With the patient in the supine position, place the probe to the right of midline transversely to the axis of the body, aiming up under the costal margin. Ask the patient to take a deep breath and tilt/fan the probe to identify the inferior vena cava, tail of caudate lobe, and portal vein dividing into right and left branches. The portal veins have characteristic hyperechoic halo/train tracks surrounding them.

INFERIOR VENA CAVA
LIVER RIGHT ATRIUM
RIGHT VENTRICLE
SUBCOSTAL
Longitudinal
FIG. 8.9

With the patient in the supine position, place the probe longitudinally oriented to the right of the midline under the right costal margin, aiming up toward the thorax. Ask the patient to take a deep breath and identify the liver speckled pattern and veins, and note inspiratory collapse

and rhythmic transmitted pulsations of the inferior vena cava. The portal vein is seen anterior to the inferior vena cava accompanied by the proper hepatic artery.

RIGHT LIVER LOBE
MORISON'S POUCH
RIGHT KIDNEY
Longitudinal
(Intercostal Oblique)
FIG. 8.10

Place the patient in the supine position and place the palm of the right hand behind the head, abducting the arm and helping to open up intercostal spaces on the right. Place the probe along the midaxillary line at about the horizontal level of the xiphisternal junction with the probe marker directed superiorly. The probe face should be rotated until it is parallel to the intercostal spaces (the intercostal oblique orientation), which minimizes rib shadowing over the structures of interest and brings the probe into closer alignment with the typical orientation of the right kidney. Identify the speckled appearance of the liver and the hyperechoic stripe representing the diaphragm over the curving superior surface of

 Figure 8.5 Subcostal longitudinal view of the left lobe of the liver, caudate lobe, the portal vein forming (from superior mesenteric vein being joined by the splenic vein), the surrounding neck and uncinate process of the pancreas, and the common hepatic artery.

173

the liver. The probe face should be tilted posteriorly until the interface between the visceral surface of the liver and the right kidney comes into view. The potential space at the hepatorenal recess is commonly referred to as Morison's pouch. This is the most dependent site in the peritoneal space above the transverse mesocolon, so it is a common location for free fluid accumulation in the upper abdomen. The hepatorenal recess should be carefully and completely scanned for any anechoic fluid collections.

Next, slide the probe superiorly (1 or 2 intercostal spaces) until the superior surface of the liver, the diaphragm, and the lower part of the right hemithorax can be seen in the image. In the presence of a normally aerated lung, the hyperechoic diaphragm creates a mirror image artifact over the lung fields such that the speckled appearance of the liver is mirrored over the right hemithorax/pleural space. The presence of free fluid in the pleural space (hemothorax or pleural effusion) abolishes the mirror image artifact and the space above the diaphragm appears anechoic, often with an atalectatic lung floating in and out of view with respiratory efforts. In addition, look carefully for any free fluid accumulation in the right subphrenic space, the potential space between the diaphragm and the superior surface of the liver.

Figure 8.6 Transverse (oblique) subcostal view of the portal triad (portal vein, proper hepatic artery, and bile duct) entering/exiting the liver via the porta hepatis. The inferior vena cava is seen immediately posterior to the portal vein. The hyperechoic falciform ligament and round ligament of the liver (ligamentum teres hepatis) are seen at the border between the left lobe of the liver (segments 2, 3) and the quadrate lobe (segment 4b).

CLINICAL APPLICATIONS

Meckel's Diverticulum

Meckel's diverticulum refers to an outpouching of the ileum. This tissue is derived from the unobliterated yolk stalk and is located 2 feet from the ileocecal junction. It is usually 2 inches in length, occurs in approximately 2% of the population, may contain 2 types of ectopic tissues (gastric and pancreatic), presents in the first 2 decades of life, and is found 2 times as frequently in boys as in girls. The diverticulum can be free or connected with the umbilicus through a fistula or a fibrous cord. Complications include ulceration, perforation, bleeding, and obstruction, which may require surgical intervention. In addition, it can mimic acute appendicitis because of similar presentation, which includes right lower quadrant abdominal pain, vomiting, and fever and should be managed surgically if it causes severe pain, significant bleeding, or obstruction.

Acute Appendicitis

Acute appendicitis refers to acute inflammation of the appendix resulting from blockage of the lumen by **fecalith** (a hard, stony mass of feces that occurs in the intestinal tract). It presents as right lower quadrant pain (McBurney's point) that starts in the periumbilical region, rebound tenderness, loss of appetite, nausea, vomiting, and fever. Rupture of the appendix can cause peritonitis leading to spread of the infection (septicemia) and death, if untreated. Appendicitis is managed surgically by appendectomy.

Liver Cirrhosis

Liver cirrhosis refers to a condition in which hepatocytes are progressively replaced by fibrous tissue surrounding the intrahepatic blood vessels and biliary radicles leading to obstruction of blood through the liver. It can be caused by chronic alcoholism; infections such as hepatitis B, C, and D; and poisons. Liver cirrhosis can result in portal hypertension, causing esophageal varices, hemorrhoids, caput medusa spider nevi or spider angioma, ascites, pedal edema, jaundice, hepatic encephalopathy, splenomegaly, hepatomegaly, palmar erythema, testicular atrophy, gynecomastia, and pectoral alopecia. Additional symptoms include fatigue, nausea, loss of appetite, and weight loss. Management includes a low-sodium and low-protein diet and diuretics. Hepatocellular carcinoma is one of the most common cancers. Risk factors include liver cirrhosis due to viral hepatitis, alcoholism, and hemochromatosis. Hepatocellular carcinoma is diagnosed based on the number of cirrhotic nodules with the liver.

Liver Biopsy

Liver biopsy is performed percutaneously under US guidance using a needle in the right eighth or ninth intercostal space at the right midaxillary line. The patient is instructed to hold their breath in full expiration to collapse the costodiaphragmatic recess, thus lessening the possibility of damage to the lung and causing pneumothorax. Transjugular liver biopsy can be performed by inserting a catheter into the internal jugular vein on the right and passing it through the superior and inferior vena cava and right hepatic vein. A needle is then inserted through the catheter to the liver and a biopsy is taken.

Fatty Liver

This term characterizes a wide array of diseases with the most common being alcoholic fatty liver disease and nonalcoholic fatty liver. Alcoholic liver disease relates to the excess of alcohol consumption, whereas nonalcoholic fatty liver relates to the insulin resistance and metabolic syndrome. In addition, viral hepatitis and certain medications can also cause triglyceride accumulation (**steatosis**). If steatosis is pronounced and chronic, it may lead to fibrosis and eventually liver cirrhosis. Recent studies place the prevalence of liver steatosis to approximately 15% of the general population. US can diagnose liver steatosis by identifying poor demarcation of intrahepatic architecture, revealing the loss of diaphragmatic demarcation, and showing that liver echogenicity is higher than that of renal cortex and spleen.

Left portal v.

Portal v.

Inferior
vena cava (IVC)

Rectus
abdominis m.

Left portal v.

Hepatic v.

Portal v.

IVC

Portal v. branch

Figure 8.7 Longitudinal (oblique) subcostal view of the portal vein approaching and entering the liver at the porta hepatis. The inferior vena cava is seen posterior to the portal vein.

Diaphragm — — Rectus abdominis m.

Right portal v. — — Left portal v.

Right lobe of liver — — Inferior vena cava (IVC)

Rectus abdominis m.

Right portal v.

Left portal v.

IVC

Right lobe of liver

Diaphragm

IVC, mirror image artifact

Figure 8.8 Transverse subcostal view of the portal vein dividing within the liver into right and left portal veins. The inferior vena cava is seen posterior to the dividing portal vein (separated by the "tail" of the caudate lobe).

Heart
(with
pericardium)

Diaphragm

Inferior
vena cava
(IVC)

Rectus
abdominis m.

Portal v.
branches

Right
ventricle

Right
atrium

Proper
hepatic a.

Portal v.

Hepatic v.

IVC

Diaphragm &
parietal pericardium

Figure 8.9 Longitudinal subcostal view of the course of the inferior vena cava posterior to the liver and approaching the right atrium (via caval hiatus of diaphragm).

Diaphragm

Right lung

Right lobe of liver

Right kidney

Intercostal mm.

Hepatorenal recess
(Morison's pouch)

Right lobe of liver

Right
kidney

Diaphragm

Right lung

Psoas major m.
& quadratus
lumborum m.

Figure 8.10 Longitudinal (intercostal oblique) view of the right hemithorax, diaphragm, right lobe of liver, Morison's pouch, and right kidney.

Gallbladder

Review of the Anatomy

The gallbladder is situated where the lateral border of rectus abdominis junctions with the right ninth costal cartilage. This is the site of **Murphy's sign**, i.e., tenderness due to acute inflammation of the gallbladder (acute cholecystitis). The gallbladder lies in a fossa between the quadrate and right lobes inferior to the liver and has a capacity of 30 to 50 m. It is located superior to the transverse colon and superolateral to the duodenum. Its structure can be divided into the neck, fundus, and body.

The neck of the gallbladder is the narrowest part and is continuous with the cystic duct, which contains spiral valves (Heister's valves). The fundus is the round blind end situated on the midclavicular line at the tip of the right ninth costal cartilage in contact with the transverse colon. The body forms the major part of the gallbladder and is in contact with the upper part of the duodenum and the transverse colon. In some cases, an abnormal conical pouch (Hartmann's pouch) might be present in the neck of the gallbladder (also known as ampulla of the gallbladder).

The gallbladder functions to receive bile, concentrate it by absorbing salts and water, store it, and release it during digestion. As the food reaches the duodenum, cholecystokinin is produced by the duodenal mucosa, which together with parasympathetic stimulation acts to contract the gallbladder, resulting in expulsion of bile into the duodenum.

The gallbladder is supplied by the cystic artery, which comes from the right hepatic artery located in the cystohepatic triangle (of Calot), formed medially by the common hepatic duct, superiorly by the visceral surface of the liver and inferiorly by the cystic duct.

Technique

GALL BLADDER
LIVER
Longitudinal
(Intercostal
Oblique)
FIG. 8.11

There are several techniques for examining the gall bladder such as subcostal, right subcostal oblique, and intercostal. However, the intercostal view uses the liver as an **insonation window** so the bowel gas does not interfere with the view. This is probably the most reliable method for learners to start with and is described as follows.

With the patient in the supine position and with the patient's right hand behind the head (this is to expand the intercostal spaces on the right side), place the probe positioned with marker side up toward right shoulder/ axilla, at the horizontal level of the xiphoid process about 7 to 8 cm lateral to xiphoid process. Align the probe with the intercostal spaces, aiming across the upper abdomen slightly posteriorly (if you tilt too far posteriorly the right kidney will come into view) to identify the anechoic lumen of the pear-shaped gall bladder. Slide the probe inferiorly to visualize as much of the gall bladder as possible. Often the bowel gas interferes with imaging the fundus, which is beyond the liver edge/costal margin. Note the veins in the liver and attempt to differentiate between hepatic veins and portal vein branches (hyperechoic halo/train tracks).

CLINICAL APPLICATIONS

Gallstones

Gallstones (cholelithiasis) are formed from crystallization of bile constituents and are made of cholesterol crystals mixed with bile pigments and calcium. Bile crystallizes to form sand, gravel, and finally stones. A common presentation of gallstones is in fat women who are fertile (multiparous) and are older than 40 years (4 F's). Stones in the fundus of the gallbladder might ulcerate through the wall of the fundus into the transverse colon passing naturally through the rectum. They might also ulcerate through the wall of the body into the duodenum and get lodged at the ileocecal junction, leading to obstruction. Stones lodged in the bile duct interfere with bile flow to the duodenum, resulting in obstructive jaundice. Finally, stones lodged at the hepatopancreatic ampulla block the biliary and the pancreatic duct systems. In this case, bile may enter the pancreatic duct system, causing aseptic or noninfectious pancreatitis.

Sonographic Murphy's Sign

Sonographic Murphy's sign refers to the subcostal view only where the probe is placed against the fundus with applied pressure. Once the patient expresses pain or maximal discomfort because of direct pressure on gallbladder only, then the sign is positive.

Figure 8.11 Intercostal (hepatic window) longitudinal view of the gallbladder.

Spleen and Kidneys

Review of the Anatomy

Spleen

The spleen is a vascular lymphatic organ located below the diaphragm at 9th to 11th ribs, i.e., at the left hypochondriac region. The spleen is supported by the splenorenal and splenogastric ligaments and is covered by the peritoneum, except at the hilum. The spleen is located superiorly to upper pole of the left kidney (almost in contact with it) and the tail of the pancreas. More specifically, the splenorenal ligament contains the splenic vessels and the tail of the pancreas.

The splenic artery supplies blood to the spleen, which empties into the splenic vein. It is divided into 2 regions, namely, the white and red pulp. The white pulp is composed of lymphatic tissue around the central arteries and is the site of phagocytic activity. The red pulp is composed of venous sinusoids and splenic cords and is the site of filtration. As the blood filters through the spleen, worn-out and damaged red blood cells and platelets are removed by macrophages. Other functions of spleen include storing blood and platelets in the red pulp, immune response, and production of mature lymphocytes, macrophages, and antibodies in the white pulp. The spleen is also the site of hematopoiesis in early life.

Kidneys

The kidneys are bilateral retroperitoneal organs located along the T12 to L3 spinal level. The right kidney is lower when compared with the contralateral left kidney because of the large size of the liver and can be found at the level of the 12th rib. The left kidney is usually found at the level of the 11th and 12th ribs. The outer layer of the kidney contains thick fibrous capsule that is enclosed by the renal fascia along with the perinephric and pararenal fat. The nerves and vessels that supply the kidney along with the ureter enter the kidney on the medial side at the hilum.

The kidney can be divided anatomically into the cortex and medulla, which contain the nephrons. The outer cortex contains the renal corpuscles and is the location of the glomerulus and the glomerular capsule (Bowman's capsule) and the proximal and distal convoluted tubules. The inner part of the kidney is the medulla and contains the loops of Henle and the collecting tubules. Several nephrons can be found in each kidney, which can be further divided into the renal corpuscle, the proximal convoluted tubule, Henle's loop, and the distal convoluted tubule.

Each kidney is supplied by the **renal artery**, which contains segmental branches with several anatomical variations, and is drained by the renal vein. Urine exits the kidney from the collecting tubules into the minor and major calyces. The major calyces empty into the renal pelvis exiting as the ureter.

Ureters

The ureter is a retroperitoneal muscular organ that joins the kidney to the urinary bladder. It courses along the iliopsoas muscle and transverse processes of the lumbar vertebrae and anterior to the bifurcation of the common iliac artery. The ureter contains certain locations where there is a high chance for **renal calculi** obstruction, which include the ureteropelvic and ureterovesicular junctions. It is supplied by branches of the abdominal aorta, renal, common and internal iliac, and gonadal arteries. Sympathetic innervation to the ureter is provided by the lumbar splanchnic nerves, whereas parasympathetic innervation is provided by the pelvic splanchnic nerves.

Adrenal Gland

The **adrenal gland** is situated at the superior medial pole of the kidney. It is a retroperitoneal organ and is invested by a capsule and the renal fascia. The adrenal gland is asymmetrical with the right adrenal gland having a pyramidal shape and the left gland having a semilunar shape. Branches from the inferior phrenic artery, the middle suprarenal artery (which is a direct branch of the aorta), and the inferior suprarenal artery (a branch of the renal artery) supply oxygenated blood to the adrenal gland. On the right, the suprarenal vein drains the gland, whereas venous drainage on the left is by the renal vein. Both venous drainage empty into the inferior vena cava.

The adrenal gland can be divided anatomically into a **cortex** and a **medulla**. The cortex has 3 separate layers, the most superficial layer being the zona glomerulosa, the middle layer the zona fasciculata, and the deepest layer the zona reticularis. Each layer of the adrenal cortex produces steroid hormones that are fundamental to maintaining homeostasis within the body. The zona glomerulosa consists of cells that produce aldosterone. The zona fasiculata cells synthesize cortisol and corticosterone. The zona reticularis secretes androgens, namely, dehydroepiandrosterone and androstenedione. The adrenal medulla has neural crest origin. The cells of the medulla are called neuroendocrine cells and play a significant role in the release of epinephrine and norepinephrine in response to sympathetic fiber stimulation.

Technique

SPLEEN
LEFT KIDNEY
Longitudinal
  (Intercostal
  Oblique)
FIG. 8.12

With the patient in the supine position or rolled into the right lateral decubitus position, place the probe with the marker pointing toward the head in the posterior axillary line (as a starting point) aligned with intercostal space. Note that decubitus positioning is not appropriate for some applications such as the focused assessment with sonography for trauma (FAST) whereby decubitus would cause fluid to drain to the right side. Fan/tilt/slide the probe, looking for grainy echotexture of the spleen as it moves with respirations. Adjust the probe to clearly see the spleen and the hyperechoic diaphragm. Then tilt to aim the beam more posteriorly (and/or slide probe posteriorly as possible) until the left kidney can be seen adjacent to the spleen (separated by potential space of splenorenal recess). Adjust position/tilt to get the best view possible of the left hemithorax, diaphragm, spleen, and left kidney. Notice that often the inferior pole of the kidney is obscured by colon gas. Observe the mirror image artifact that causes the appearance of the spleen echotexture in the left pleural space (abolished by free fluid such as hemothorax or left pleural effusion). Place the patient in a right lateral decubitus position if there is substantial bowel gas shadowing.

LEFT KIDNEY
Longitudinal
  (Intercostal
  Oblique)
FIG. 8.13

Position the patient and the probe as shown in Figure 8.12. Slide the probe as far posteriorly as possible (it is already near the examination table surface) and adjust the tilt/angle/position to image as much of the left kidney as possible. It may be necessary to gently roll the patient into the right decubitus position to position the probe behind the posterior axillary line and image the kidney from posterior to the left colic flexure (gas shadowing), identifying the cortex and columns, renal pyramids, hyperechoic fat, and connective tissue of the renal sinus.

SPLEEN
Longitudinal
  (Intercostal
  Oblique)
FIG. 8.14

Position the patient and the probe as shown in Figure 8.12. Slide the probe superiorly and aim the beam slightly anteriorly to image the spleen in its long axis,

| Figure 8.12 | Longitudinal (intercostal oblique) view of the left hemithorax, spleen, and left kidney. |

Figure 8.13 Longitudinal (intercostal oblique) view of the left kidney.

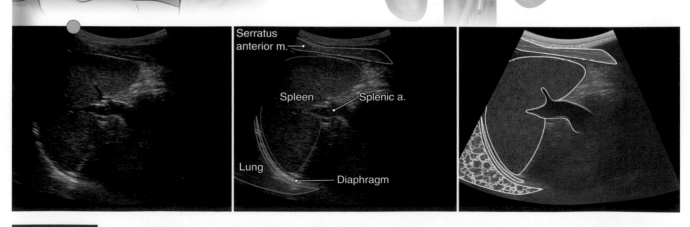

Figure 8.14 Longitudinal (intercostal oblique) view of the spleen.

observing its hyperechoic grainy echotexture, the hyperechoic diaphragm along its superior surface, and respiratory movements of the spleen and diaphragm.

RIGHT KIDNEY
Longitudinal
(Intercostal
Oblique)
FIG. 8.15

With the patient in the supine position, place the probe midaxillary line approximately at the level of the xiphisternal junction, aligned with an intercostal space to minimize rib shadowing. Aim slightly posteriorly (toward the spine) to view the liver, the hepatorenal recess, and the right kidney. Slide the probe inferiorly (and realign with the intercostal space) until the right kidney can be seen from the superior pole to the inferior pole (gas shadowing may interfere with imaging of the inferior pole beyond the inferior edge of the right liver lobe). Identify Morison's pouch, kidney capsule, psoas muscles, and vertebral bodies. A subcostal approach is also used to identify the kidney to avoid bowel gas by using the liver as an insonation window.

CLINICAL APPLICATIONS

Splenomegaly is the result of venous congestion due to portal hypertension or thrombosis of the splenic vein. It typically leads to sequestration of blood resulting in thrombocytopenia and easy bruising. Its symptoms include weight loss, night sweats, fever, diarrhea, and bone pain.

Splenic rupture most commonly occurs because of fractured ribs or severe trauma in the left hypochondrium, leading to severe bleeding. It is difficult to surgically repair a ruptured spleen, and splenectomy is performed to prevent death due to exsanguination. The spleen can be removed, as its functions are assumed by other reticuloendothelial organs.

Cancer of the lymphoid tissue is called **lymphoma**. **Hodgkin's disease** is a type of malignant lymphoma, and its clinical features include painless, progressive enlargement of the lymph nodes, spleen, and other lymphoid tissue; night sweats; fever; and weight loss.

Urolithiasis is the condition in which renal calculi may present at any part of the urinary tract. About 70% to 80% of kidney stones (renal calculus or nephrolith) are formed of high levels of calcium and, as a result, are easily detectable with US when patients are suspected for nephrolithiasis because of renal colic. Based on the size and shape of kidney stones, severe colicky pain may be produced at the renal calyx or while traveling down through the ureter. In addition, hydronephrosis or obstruction of the ureters by a stone can be a surgical emergency. Another type of kidney stone is the Staghorn calculi or coral calculi. These stones fill every part of the renal pelvis and calyces. Their composition is of magnesium ammonium phosphate, known as struvite, or calcium carbonate apatite. They are formed most commonly in women owing to recurrent infections. The clinical symptoms include fever, pain, hematuria, and abscess formation.

Figure 8.15 Longitudinal (intercostal oblique) view of the right kidney and right liver lobe.

Pancreas

Review of the Anatomy

The pancreas is located on the floor of the lesser sac in the left hypochondriac and epigastric regions, forming a portion of the bed of the stomach. It is situated in the retroperitoneal space, except a small portion of its tail, which is located in the splenorenal ligament. The head of the pancreas is situated in the C-shaped curvature of the duodenum. The uncinate process of the pancreas is the lower part of its head located to the left posterior to the superior mesenteric vessels. It is an exocrine gland that produces digestive enzymes involved in fat, protein, and carbohydrate digestion and an endocrine gland (islets of Langerhans), because it secretes insulin and glucagon, which are involved in the metabolism of glucose.

The blood supply of the pancreas is from branches of the splenic artery and the inferior and superior pancreaticoduodenal arteries. The pancreas consists of 2 ducts, the main pancreatic duct and the accessory pancreatic duct.

The main pancreatic duct (duct of Wirsung) starts in the tail, courses to the right along the pancreas, and drains pancreatic juice, which contains enzymes. The bile duct and the main pancreatic duct join to form the hepatopancreatic ampulla (ampulla of Vater) as it enters the second part of the duodenum at the greater papilla. The accessory pancreatic duct (Santorini's duct) starts in the lower part of the head of the pancreas to drain a portion of the body and head. It eventually empties at the lesser duodenal papilla superior to the greater papilla.

Technique

PANCREAS
ABDOMINAL AORTA
Longitudinal
  (Parasagittal)
FIG. 8.16

With the patient in the supine position, place the probe in the longitudinal axis of the body just left of midline. You may need to start high in the epigastric area and slide inferiorly while applying pressure to the probe face to move bowel gas. Ask the patient to take a deep breath (asking patient to drink a water load of 2 or 3 glasses may improve imaging by displacing stomach gas) while you identify the left lobe of the liver and its edges and contours. Tilt the probe to identify the pulsations of the abdominal aorta and adjust the beam angle until the aorta is roughly horizontal (rather than curving steeply up inferiorly with the lumbar curvature). Identify the celiac and superior mesenteric branches of the aorta. Anterior to the proximal part of superior mesenteric artery, locate the splenic vein posterior to the body of the pancreas. The pancreas echo texture is variable but generally similar to the liver with a slightly hypoechoic background with hyperechoic speckling. The left renal vein may be visible (physiologically compressed) in the space between the superior mesenteric artery and the anterior surface of the abdominal aorta.

HEAD OF PANCREAS
UNCINATE PROCESS
NECK OF PANCREAS
BODY OF PANCREAS
Transverse
FIG. 8.17

With the patient in the supine position, place the probe transversely across the midline. You may need to start high in the epigastric area and slide inferiorly applying pressure to the probe face to move bowel gas. Ask the patient to take a deep breath (asking patient to drink a water load of 2 or 3 glasses may improve imaging by displacing stomach gas).

| **Figure 8.16** | Longitudinal (parasagittal) view of the body of the pancreas in relationship to the left liver lobe, splenic vein, and abdominal aorta with its celiac and superior mesenteric branches. |

With the probe in a transverse position across the midline, adjust the angle/tilt to look for the echotexture of the pancreas posterior to the left lobe of the liver lobe and, more importantly, in relationship to abdominal vessels such as superior mesenteric and splenic veins at its posterior surface. Look for the superior mesenteric artery to the left of the superior mesenteric vein with a hyperechoic ring (surrounded by fat and connective tissue at the root of the mesentery), the head of the pancreas to the right of the superior mesenteric vein with uncinate process extending posterior to the superior mesenteric vein, a pulsating aorta just along the left side of the vertebral body, and a left renal vein in the space between the aorta and the superior mesenteric artery (physiologically compressed in the space and expanding beyond) leading to the inferior vena cava to the right of the vertebral body. The neck of the pancreas is situated anterior to superior mesenteric vessels and the body extends posteriorly out of view beyond the superior mesenteric vessels.

CLINICAL APPLICATIONS

Pancreatitis refers to inflammation of the pancreas and can be caused by gallstones or alcohol consumption. Its symptoms include severe and constant epigastric pain radiating to the back.

Pancreatic cancer can present as severe back pain and can invade into the surrounding organs. It usually presents late and thus is difficult to treat. Surgical resection called a pancreaticoduodenectomy (Whipple's procedure) is possible in some cases. Cancer of the head can compress the bile duct, leading to obstructive jaundice. Cancer of the neck and body can cause obstruction of the portal vein or inferior vena cava as the pancreas is in proximity to these veins.

 Transverse view of pancreas along with superior mesenteric artery and vein, splenic vein, left renal vein, inferior vena cava, and aorta.

Abdominal Vessels

Review of the Anatomy

Celiac and Mesenteric Arteries

The celiac trunk is a branch from the abdominal aorta, located at the anterior surface of the aorta just below the aortic hiatus of the diaphragm. The celiac trunk trifurcates into the left gastric, splenic, and common hepatic arteries.

The smallest branch from the celiac trunk is the left gastric artery. The left gastric artery travels superiorly toward the gastric cardia and communicates to the esophagus and liver with branches to the esophageal and hepatic arteries. The left gastric artery also runs along the lesser curvature of the stomach forming a connection with the right gastric artery.

The splenic artery is a large, tortuous vessel that courses over the superior surface of the pancreas before entering the splenoreal ligament. This artery is the largest branch of the celiac trunk and usually has numerous terminal branches that include the short gastric arteries, the left gastroepiploic (gastro-omental) artery, and pancreatic branches.

The short gastric arteries supply the fundus of the stomach and course through the splenogastric ligament. The left gastroepiploic artery supplies the stomach and greater omentum by also passing through the splenogastric ligament to reach the greater omentum and course beside the greater curvature of the stomach. One of the pancreatic vessels, which branches off the splenic artery, includes the dorsal pancreatic artery.

After arising from the celiac trunk the common hepatic artery travels toward the liver along the superior border of the pancreas. The common hepatic artery will branch into the proper hepatic artery, the gastroduodenal artery, and occasionally the right gastric artery. The proper hepatic artery is located along the free edge of the lesser omentum. The proper hepatic artery divides into the left and right hepatic arteries. The right hepatic artery subsequently divides into the cystic artery at the cystohepatic triangle of Calot. The borders of the triangle of Calot are the cystic duct, the common hepatic duct, and the inferior border of the liver. The right gastric artery can arise from the common hepatic artery, but occasionally the artery may originate from the proper hepatic artery. The right gastric artery travels to the pylorus of the stomach and along the lesser

curvature of the stomach where it forms an anastomosis with the left gastric artery. The gastroduodenal artery travels posterior to the first part of the duodenum. It is known to give off multiple branches, including the supraduodenal artery superiorly and various retroduodenal arteries inferiorly. In particular, the gastroduodenal artery divides into the right gastroepiploic artery and the superior pancreaticoduodenal artery.

The right gastroepiploic artery travels along the greater curvature of the stomach. It provides blood supply to the stomach and the greater omentum. The superior pancreaticoduodenal artery courses between the head of the pancreas and the duodenum. The superior pancreaticoduodenal artery divides into the anterior-superior pancreaticoduodenal artery and the posterior-superior pancreaticoduodenal artery.

Superior Mesenteric Artery

The superior mesenteric artery arises from the abdominal aorta posterior to the neck of the pancreas. It descends behind the uncinate process of the pancreas and the third part of the duodenum and enters the root of the mesentery posterior to the transverse colon and runs in the right iliac fossa. The superior mesenteric artery gives rise to 5 terminal branches: the inferior pancreaticoduodenal artery, the middle colic artery, the right colic artery, the ileocolic artery, and the intestinal arteries. The inferior pancreatoduodenal artery courses to the right and divides into 2 branches, the anterior-inferior pancreaticoduodenal artery and the posterior-inferior pancreaticoduodenal artery. The inferior pancreaticoduodenal artery (anterior and posterior) will then anastomose with respective branches of the superior pancreaticoduodenal artery.

The middle colic artery bifurcates into the right and left branches. The right branch anastomoses with the right colic artery, and the left branch also has connections with the ascending branch of the left colic artery. As these arterial connections occur, the marginal artery forms running along the large bowel.

The right colic artery originates from the superior mesenteric artery and courses to the right behind the peritoneum. The right colic artery may frequently arise from the ileocolic artery. The right colic artery terminates into ascending and descending branches, which course along the ascending colon.

The ileocolic artery traverses inferiorly, posterior to the peritoneum toward the right iliac fossa. It then divides into the ascending colic artery, anterior and posterior cecal arteries, the appendicular artery, and ileal branches. The ascending colic artery forms an anastomosis with the right colic artery. Branches from the superior mesenteric artery (usually 12-15 in number) supply the jejunum and ileum. The intestinal arteries branch and anastomose to form a series of arcades in the mesentery.

Inferior Mesenteric Artery

The inferior mesenteric artery arises inferiorly to the superior mesenteric artery on the anterior surface of the aorta and courses to the left posterior to the peritoneum. Terminal branches of the inferior mesenteric artery supplies the descending colon, the sigmoid colon, and the upper portion of the rectum. The inferior mesenteric artery trifurcates into the left colic artery, the sigmoid artery, and the superior rectal artery. The left colic artery courses to the left toward the descending colon and normally divides into ascending and descending branches. The sigmoid arteries (2-3 in number) course toward the sigmoid colon in its mesentery dividing into ascending and descending branches. The superior rectal artery descends into the pelvis and terminates into 2 branches. The branches of the superior rectal artery course along the sides of the rectum and will connect with the middle and inferior rectal arteries.

Veins

Portal Vein

The **portal vein** is formed by the splenic vein and the superior mesenteric vein posterior to the neck of the pancreas. The portal vein is about 8 cm (3.2 in.) long and collects venous blood from the abdominal part of the gut, spleen, pancreas, and gallbladder.

Inferior Mesenteric Vein

The inferior mesenteric vein does not directly drain into the portal vein. The inferior mesenteric vein can merge with the splenic or the superior mesenteric vein or at the junction of these 2 veins. The inferior mesenteric also receives venous drainage from the left gastric (or coronary) vein. This vein courses superiorly behind the bile duct and

hepatic artery within the free margin of the lesser omentum, carrying deoxygenated blood and nutrients extracted from digestion. It carries 3 times as much blood as the hepatic artery and has a higher blood pressure than in the inferior vena cava.

Superior Mesenteric Vein

The superior mesenteric vein courses along the right side of the superior mesenteric artery. Some of the branches of the superior mesenteric vein also follow the tributaries of the superior mesenteric artery. The root of the superior mesenteric vein usually traverses the third part of the duodenum and the uncinate process of the pancreas. The termination of the superior mesenteric vein is located behind the neck of the pancreas. At this point the splenic vein merges with the superior mesenteric vein to form the portal vein.

Splenic Vein

The splenic vein (formerly known as the lineal vein) originates from the merging of venous sinusoids in the spleen. The splenic vein also receives venous drainage from the short gastric, left gastroepiploic, and pancreatic veins.

Inferior Mesenteric Vein

The inferior mesenteric veins originate from the joining of the superior rectal and sigmoid veins. The inferior mesenteric vein receives venous drainage from the left colic vein. Often the inferior mesenteric vein will drain into the splenic vein. However, the inferior mesenteric vein can drain directly into the superior mesenteric vein or at the merging point of the superior mesenteric vein and splenic vein.

Left Gastric (Coronary) Vein

The left gastric (coronary) vein usually spans over a short distance in the superior portion of the lesser curvature of the stomach, where it is nestled between the 2 lesser omental layers. The left gastric vein continues to travel toward the junction of the stomach and esophagus. At this point the left gastric vein can join venous tributaries of the esophagus, which eventually empty into the azygous vein, thus formulating the systemic venous distribution of the left gastric vein. In addition, the left gastric vein drains into the portal vein directly as well as through an anastomosis with the right gastric vein, to form the portal venous portion of the left gastric vein.

Paraumbilical Veins

The paraumbilical veins are nested in the falciform ligament. These veins connect the left branch of the portal vein with small periumbilical subcutaneous veins. The periumbilical subcutaneous veins are radicles of the superior epigastric, inferior epigastric, thoracoepigastric, and superficial epigastric veins. The paraumbilical veins are almost always closed but can become patent and dilated in portal hypertension.

Hepatic Veins

The hepatic veins (left, right, and middle) are valveless veins located in the intersegmental planes of the liver. These veins drain into the inferior vena cava; however, frequently the left and middle hepatic vein often merge before joining the inferior vena cava.

Technique

AORTA
CELIAC ARTERY
SUPERIOR
    MESENTERIC
    ARTERY
Longitudinal
   (Parasagittal)
FIG. 8.18

With the patient in the supine position, place the probe in the longitudinal axis of the body just left of midline. You may need to start high in epigastric area and slide inferiorly, applying pressure to the probe face to move bowel gas. Ask the patient to take a deep breath (asking patient to drink a water load of 2 or 3 glasses may improve imaging by displacing stomach gas). Identify the left lobe of the liver and its edges and contours.

Tilt the probe face to identify the pulsations of the abdominal aorta and adjust the beam angle until the aorta is roughly horizontal (rather than curving steeply up inferiorly with the lumbar curvature). Identify the celiac and superior mesenteric branches of the aorta. Anterior to the proximal part of superior mesenteric artery, locate the splenic vein posteriorly to the body of the pancreas. The pancreas echo texture is variable but generally similar to the liver, slightly hypoechoic background with hyperechoic speckling. The left renal vein may be visible (physiologically compressed) in the space between the superior mesenteric artery and the anterior surface of the abdominal aorta.

CELIAC ARTERY
SPLENIC ARTERY
COMMON HEPATIC
    BRANCHES
Transverse
FIG. 8.19

With the patient in the supine position, place the probe transversely with the marker pointing to the right. Identify the left lobe of the liver and the bodies of the lumbar vertebrae. Identify the aorta and inferior vena cava along the vertebral body. Slide the probe and tilt/fan while watching for the celiac artery and the sweeping "gull-wing" appearance of its splenic and common hepatic branches.

Figure 8.18   Longitudinal (parasagittal) view of the abdominal aorta along with its celiac and superior mesenteric branches.

The splenic artery is useful for "following" along the body of the pancreas. The portal vein is seen immediately anterior to the inferior vena cava.

> **SUPERIOR MESENTERIC ARTERY**
> **SUPERIOR MESENTERIC VEIN**
> **AORTA**
> **INFERIOR VENA CAVA**
> Transverse
> **FIG. 8.20**

Continue from Figure 8.19 and tilt/fan and slide slightly inferiorly while watching for the next ventral branch of the aorta, the superior mesenteric artery. The celiac and the superior mesenteric branches of the aorta arise very close together, and only slight movements (sliding/tilting) of the probe go back and forth between them. After identifying the superior mesenteric artery, adjust the probe position until the superior mesenteric artery can be clearly seen surrounded by a hyperechoic ring (of fat/connective tissue at the root of the mesentery) just to the left of the superior mesenteric vein. Tilt/slide up and down to see the splenic vein joining the superior mesenteric vein from the left side, forming the portal vein behind the neck of the pancreas (superior to the position

where the splenic vein joins the superior mesenteric vein is the portal vein). Look for the echotexture and identify the pancreatic head and uncinate process adjacent to the superior mesenteric vein. Carefully adjust the position of the probe to identify the right renal artery and the (physiologically compressed) left renal vein traversing the space between the superior mesenteric vein and aorta to join the inferior vena cava. In this image, the falciform ligament is clearly seen at the border between the left liver lobe and quadrate lobe. The right crus of the diaphragm is also well seen in this image along the vertebral body, between the inferior vena cava and aorta.

> **SUPERIOR MESENTERIC VESSELS**
> **SPLENIC VEIN**
> **AORTA**
> **INFERIOR VENA CAVA**
> Transverse
> **FIG. 8.21**

Place the probe in the same position as in Figure 8.20 and adjust the probe position to see the splenic vein joining the superior mesenteric vein. Keep as much of the splenic vein in view as possible. Follow the body of the pancreas to the left and posteriorly, and identify the superior

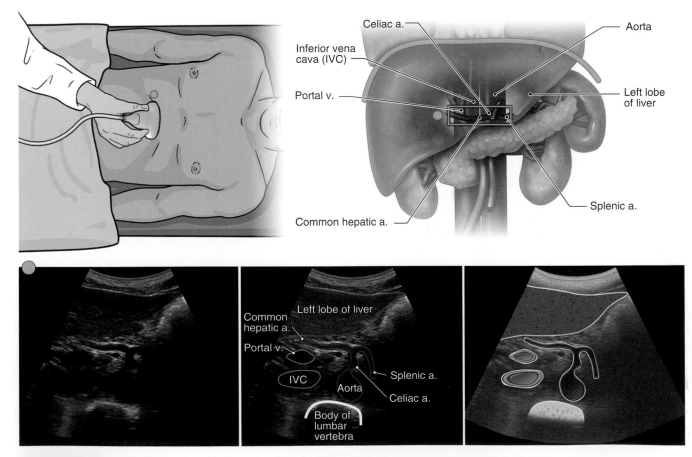

Figure 8.19 Transverse view of the celiac artery along with its splenic and common hepatic branches.

mesenteric vessels, the aorta, the inferior vena cava, and their relationships with the left renal vein.

ABDOMINAL AORTA INFERIOR VENA CAVA
Transverse
FIG. 8.22

Starting from the superior mesenteric artery in Figure 8.21, slide the probe inferiorly keeping the aorta and inferior vena cava in view to a position a few centimeters above the umbilicus. The bifurcation of the abdominal aorta occurs approximately at the level of the umbilicus. The aorta and inferior vena cava become progressively more superficial inferiorly, following the lumbar curvature of the spine. There is small intestine and gas shadowing, but as the vessels and the lumbar vertebrae become more superficial, it becomes fairly easy to apply probe pressure to gently push intestinal gas out of the way.

BIFURCATION OF ABDOMINAL AORTA
Transverse
FIG. 8.23

Continue from Figure 8.22 and follow the aorta inferiorly to about the level of the umbilicus (need to fill the umbilicus with gel to eliminate air shadowing and poor image quality when the probe is over the umbilicus). At this level the aorta typically divides into the right and left common iliac arteries. After identifying the right and left common iliac arteries at their origin, slide the probe a few centimeters inferiorly and observe the left common iliac vein crossing horizontally behind the iliac arteries to join the more vertical right common iliac vein at the confluence of the inferior vena cava.

INFERIOR VENA CAVA
Longitudinal (Subcostal)
FIG. 8.24

With the patient in the supine position, place the probe in the longitudinal axis of the body just right of the midline under the right costal margin, aimed up toward the thorax (a deep breath by the patient may be helpful). Identify the liver speckled pattern and veins; note inspiratory collapse and rhythmic transmitted pulsations of the inferior vena cava. The portal vein is seen anterior to the inferior vena cava, accompanied by the proper hepatic artery.

Superior mesenteric v. (SMV)

Head of pancreas

Uncinate process of pancreas

Inferior vena cava (IVC)

Superior mesenteric a. (SMA)

Left renal v.

Aorta

Right renal a.

Rectus abdominis m.

Falciform lig.

L. lobe of liver

Quadrate lobe of liver

Pancreas

SMV

SMA

IVC

Aorta

L. renal v.

R. renal a.

R. crus of diaphragm

Body of lumbar vertebra

 Figure 8.20 Transverse view of the superior mesenteric artery and vein, head and uncinate process of the pancreas, abdominal aorta, and inferior vena cava.

8 Abdomen

CLINICAL APPLICATIONS

Abdominal Aortic Aneurysm

Abdominal aortic aneurysm is defined as the dilatations of the abdominal aorta if greater than 50% of its proximal normal segment (>3 cm). Men are more commonly affected, and it is present in approximately 10% of the population over 65 years of age. Unfortunately, the majority of abdominal aortic aneurysms are asymptomatic and are diagnosed incidentally during routine examinations. However, the most common complication of abdominal aortic aneurysm is rupture, which presents with severe abdominal pain or back pain leading to hypovolemic shock with a high mortality rate. The most common causes leading to aneurysm are atherosclerosis, inflammation, chronic aortic dissection, different types of vasculitis, and Marfan and Ehler-Danlos syndromes.

Splenic Artery Aneurysm

Splenic artery aneurysm is the most common aneurysm of the viscera. These focal dilatations of the splenic artery can be saccular or true aneurysms. These aneurysms are more common in women; however, rupture is more common in men. Their discovery is typically incidental, but they are most commonly associated with atherosclerosis, different types of vasculitis, fibromuscular dysplasia, portal hypertension, and cirrhosis. The most common complication of splenic aneurysm is rupture (5% of cases), which presents with left upper quadrant pain. There is a double-rupture sign when the initial blood after the rupture collects at the lesser sac and provides a pseudohemodynamic stabilization, followed by sudden hypovolemic shock when the blood moves into the peritoneal cavity.

Figure 8.21 Transverse view of the superior mesenteric artery and vein, head, uncinate process, neck and body of the pancreas, splenic vein, abdominal aorta, and inferior vena cava.

198

Inferior vena cava (IVC)

Psoas major m.

Body of lumbar vertebra

Rectus abdominis m.

Small intestine

Aorta

Rectus abdominis m.

Small intestine

Aorta

IVC

Psoas major m.

Body of lumbar vertebra

Psoas major m.

Figure 8.22 Transverse view, above the umbilicus, of the aorta and inferior vena cava in relationship to lumbar vertebral body and psoas major muscles.

Rectus abdominis m.

Small intestine

Right common iliac a.

Left common iliac a.

Psoas major m.

Body of lumbar vertebra

Inferior vena cava (IVC)

Rectus abdominis m.

R. & L. common iliac a.

Small intestine

IVC

Body of lumbar vertebra

Psoas major m.

Psoas major m.

Figure 8.23 Transverse view of the bifurcation of the abdominal aorta into right and left common iliac arteries.

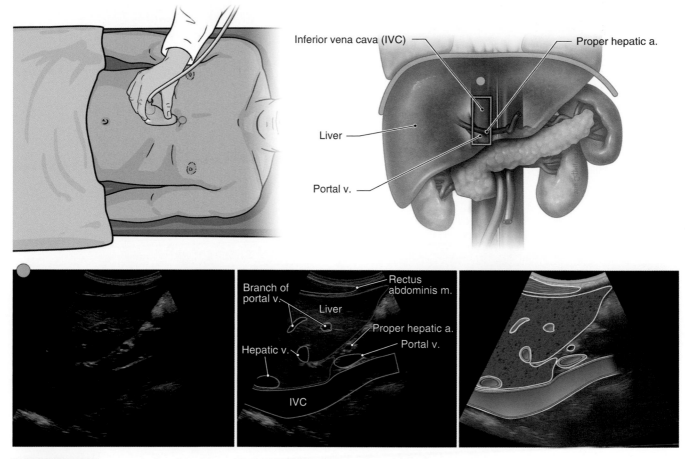

Figure 8.24 Longitudinal (subcostal) view of the course of the inferior vena cava posterior to the liver.

9

Neck, Face, Eye

Neck

Review of the Anatomy

The neck is a compact region that is an intersection between the head, thorax, and upper limb. Geometrically, the neck classically has been divided into multiple triangles to aid in the study of its anatomy. Although not all of these triangles are used clinically, some are useful for descriptive purposes. We will divide and describe the major structures of the neck by considering the anatomy within the posterior and anterior cervical triangles. The nuchal or posterior aspect of the neck will not be considered in this description.

Fasciae

The fasciae of the neck can be simplified into 2 layers.

1. *Superficial cervical fascia:* This layer is located in a subcutaneous location.
2. *Deep cervical fascia:* These fasciae subdivide the deeper layers of the neck. Each of these layers contributes to the column of fascia known as the carotid sheath, which envelopes the carotid artery, internal jugular vein, and vagus nerve in the neck.

Superficial investing envelopes the outer perimeter of the neck splitting to encase the sternocleidomastoid and trapezius muscles. *Prevertebral* covers the cervical vertebrae and their attached muscles such as the longus and scalene muscles. *Pretracheal* and *buccopharyngeal layers* surround the larynx/trachea, thyroid gland, and pharynx/esophagus. Primarily for convenience of description, the neck is divided into various triangles. We will focus on the 2 larger divisions, the posterior and anterior triangles and their contents.

Posterior Cervical Triangle

The posterior cervical triangle is bounded interiorly by the posterior edge of the sternocleidomastoid, posteriorly by the anterior edge of the upper trapezius, and inferiorly by the middle third of the clavicle.

The roof of this geometric region is the investing layer of deep cervical fascia and part of the platysma muscle as it travels from the mandible to the fascia over the pectoralis major and deltoid muscles. The muscular floor of this triangle covered by prevertebral fascia is composed of from anterior to posterior the scalenes, the levator scapulae, the splenius capitis, and a small portion of the semispinalis

capitis. The inferior belly of the omohyoid muscle also crosses superficial to these aforementioned muscles on its way from the scapula to the hyoid bone. The inferior belly of the omohyoid divides the posterior cervical triangle into an upper occipital and a lower subclavian triangle. In addition, the small upper portion of the serratus anterior muscle is found here. Lastly, the spinal accessory nerve, the posterior lymphatic chain, and the emergence of brachial plexus are found in this triangle.

Muscles

The following muscles are located in the posterior cervical triangle:

- **Trapezius:** This muscle arises from the midline from near the external occipital protuberance, along the spinous processes and associated ligaments inferiorly to the 12th thoracic vertebrae. This muscle then travels laterally to attach to the scapula and lateral clavicle. Its upper fibers elevate the scapula.
- **Sternocleidomastoid:** This muscle arises from the manubrium of the sternum and medial aspect of the clavicle. This muscle then ascends to attach to the mastoid process of the temporal bone.
- **Scalenes:** These muscles arise from the cervical vertebrae and descend to attach to the first and second ribs. Functionally, the scalene muscles (anterior, middle, and posterior) are used to elevate the first and second ribs as is seen in forced inspiration.
- **Levator scapulae:** This muscle attaches medially to the transverse processes of the upper 4 cervical vertebrae and laterally to the superior angle of the scapula. On contraction, this muscle elevates and retracts the scapula.
- **Splenius capitis:** This muscle originates from the spinous processes and associated ligaments of the cervical and upper thoracic spinous processes and travels superiorly to insert onto the mastoid process and superior nuchal line. Bilateral contraction results in extension of the neck.
- **Semispinalis capitis:** This muscle attaches superiorly between the superior and inferior nuchal lines and inferiorly from the transverse and articular processes and associated ligaments of the lower cervical and upper thoracic vertebrae.

- **Serratus anterior:** This muscle arises typically from the upper 8 ribs and inserts onto the vertebral border of the scapula.

Vessels

The major blood vessels of the posterior triangle are the subclavian artery and vein. The subclavian artery as it crosses over the first rib lies between the anterior and middle scalene muscles. The subclavian vein, however, travels just anterior to the anterior scalene muscle.

Lymphatics

Lymphatics, including nodes, are found scattered throughout the posterior cervical triangle, including along the superficially located accessory nerve (see following text). At the base of the posterior cervical triangle (e.g., middle third of the clavicle), the lower deep cervical lymph nodes traveling with the internal jugular vein are referred to as the supraclavicular nodes of Virchow and, if enlarged, may signal malignancies of the viscera.

Nerves

Cutaneous Nerves

Four cutaneous nerves derived from the cervical plexus (C1–C4) emanate from the posterior border of the sternocleidomastoid muscle at a so-called nerve point found at the junction of the upper third and lower two-thirds of this muscle.

- **Lesser occipital nerve:** This branch, derived from C2 and C3, ascends along the posterior border of the sternocleidomastoid toward the skin of the auricle and occiput.
- **Great auricular nerve:** This nerve, derived from C2 and C3, ascends superficial to this muscle toward the ear and skin over the parotid region.
- **Transverse cervical nerve:** This nerve, derived from C2 and C3, travels anteriorly and superficial to the sternocleidomastoid toward the midline of the neck.
- **Supraclavicular nerve:** This branch, derived from C3 and C4, travels inferiorly and terminates as 3 branches that cross the medial, middle, and lateral aspects of the clavicle to supply regional skin.

Accessory Nerve

One important superficial nerve of the posterior triangle is the accessory nerve or the 11th cranial nerve. This nerve innervates only 2 muscles in the body, the sternocleidomastoid and trapezius muscles. After innervating the deep surface of the sternocleidomastoid muscle, the accessory nerve emerges from the posterior border of this muscle at approximately the junction between its upper third and lower two-thirds and then descends to the trapezius muscle just superficial to the levator scapulae muscle.

Brachial Plexus

The proximal parts (rami and trunks) of the brachial plexus formed by ventral rami of C5 to T1 are found in the posterior cervical triangle and are bordered by the anterior and middle scalene muscles. Between these 2 muscles, the proximal brachial plexus is just posterior to the subclavian artery.

Phrenic Nerve

In the neck, the phrenic nerve (C3, C4, and C5), which supplies the diaphragm, descends almost vertically along the superficial surface of the anterior scalene muscle to travel between the subclavian artery and vein. Injury to this nerve may impair respiration. Irritation of this nerve results in spasm of the ipsilateral diaphragm (e.g., hiccups).

C3 and C4

Branches of C3 and C4 may also travel through the posterior cervical triangle to terminate in the trapezius muscle or communicate with the accessory nerve. These nerves can be motor to the trapezius; however, the exact nature of such branches is debated.

Dorsal Scapular Nerve

This proximal branch of the C5 contribution to the brachial plexus exits the middle scalene muscle and travels posteriorly to the rhomboid muscles and sometimes the levator scapulae.

Long Thoracic Nerve

Either a portion or the entire long thoracic nerve, which arises from the upper 3 rami contributing to the brachial plexus, exits the middle scalene muscle to travel anteroinferiorly to terminate in the serratus anterior muscle.

Anterior Cervical Triangle

The anterior cervical triangle contains not only the main blood supply for the head but also many cranial nerves and viscera such as the larynx and thyroid gland. The topography of the anterior cervical triangle includes:

- **Hyoid:** This U-shaped bone composed of a body and greater and lesser horns (cornu) does not articulate to surrounding bones but is rather suspended by muscles and ligaments at the C3 vertebral level. Its greater and lesser horns allow for attachment of muscles and ligaments.

- **Thyroid cartilage:** The thyroid cartilage is one of the 9 cartilages of the larynx and the largest of these. This structure sits anterior to the C4 and C5 vertebrae. The thyroid cartilage is connected superiorly to the hyoid bone via the thyrohyoid membrane and inferiorly to the cricoid cartilage by the cricothyroid ligament.
- **Cricoid cartilage:** This ring-shaped cartilage of the larynx lies anterior to the sixth cervical vertebrae and marks the transition from larynx to trachea and pharynx to esophagus.

Muscles

The anterior cervical triangle is bordered by the anterior aspect of the sternocleidomastoid and the lower border of the mandible and the midline. Conveniently, muscles of the anterior cervical triangle can be generally divided into those that are superior to and those that are inferior to the hyoid bone. The infrahyoid muscles include from lateral to medial the omohyoid (discussed earlier), the sternohyoid, the sternothyroid and thyrohyoid, and the cricothyroid. These muscles are named for their connections inferosuperiorly and, in general, assist in the movement of the hyoid bone and thyroid cartilage, which is one of the 9 cartilages of the larynx (voice box). These muscles may also assist in depressing the mandible. The cricothyroid is a muscle of the larynx that modifies the pitch of the voice. The very thin platysma muscle covers these muscles in its descent from the lower jaw to the fascia of the pectoral and deltoid regions.

Suprahyoid muscles include the anterior and posterior bellies of the digastric, the mylohyoid, geniohyoid, stylohyoid, and hyoglossus. Each of these muscles, as many of their names imply, have some connection to the hyoid bone. The digastric muscle arises from the temporal bone (posterior belly) and inserts onto the mandible (anterior belly). An intermediate tendon connects these 2 bellies and is tethered to the hyoid bone by a thickening of fascia. The mylohyoid and geniohyoid arise from the internal aspect of the mandible and the stylohyoid from the styloid process of the temporal bone. The hyoglossus arises from the lateral aspect of the hyoid bone and inserts into the tongue. This muscle depresses the tongue within the oral cavity. Collectively, these muscles help to elevate the hyoid bone and indirectly attached larynx. The mylohyoid muscle serves as the main component of the floor of the oral cavity.

A deeper group of muscles are located over the anterior aspect of the vertebral column and are together referred to as the prevertebral muscles. These include the scalenes (discussed earlier), the longus cervicis, and longus capitis muscles. These muscles together help flex the cervical spine and craniocervical junction.

Nerves

Cervical Branch of the Facial Nerve

This small branch of cranial nerve VII supplies the platysma muscle.

Cervical Plexus

The cervical plexus is composed of fibers from the first 4 cervical ventral rami and includes cutaneous branches (described earlier in the posterior cervical triangle)—the ansa cervicalis, the phrenic nerve (described earlier), branches to the accessory nerve from C2 to C4 (described earlier), and direct muscular branches to the prevertebral muscles.

Ansa Cervicalis

Fibers from C1 to C3 unite and form a loop known as the ansa cervicalis that normally courses just anterior to the internal jugular vein. The superior root formed by C1 and C2 fibers that run with the hypoglossal nerve and the inferior root is derived from the second and third cervical nerves. This motor nerve supplies the infrahyoid muscles. A branch of C1 innervates the thyrohyoid and geniohyoid muscles by traveling along the hypoglossal nerve.

C2 and C3

These branches may also innervate the sternocleidomastoid muscle and, as the C3 and C4 fibers that terminate in the trapezius muscle, have an equivocal function.

Cervical Branches to the Scalenes and Prevertebral Muscles

Proximal branches from the ventral rami of cervical spinal nerves innervate the anterior, middle, and posterior scalenes, as well as the longus cervicis and capitis and rectus capitis and lateralis muscles.

Nerve to Mylohyoid

A branch of the third division (V3) of the trigeminal nerve (cranial nerve V) or mandibular nerve innervates the mylohyoid and anterior belly of the digastric muscle and is therefore known as the nerve to the mylohyoid.

Vagus Nerve

In the neck, the vagus nerve has several branches. These include a pharyngeal nerve that supplies all muscles of the pharynx and soft palate and a superior laryngeal nerve that divides into an internal and external branch. The internal branch is a sensory nerve to the mucosa of the larynx superior to the vocal cords, and the external branch supplies primarily the cricothyroid muscle. The recurrent laryngeal nerves ascend symmetrically in a groove between the trachea and esophagus but have different courses inferiorly between the left and right sides. On the left side, this nerve loops around the aortic arch, and on the right side, it loops more proximally around the subclavian artery. Other branches of the vagus nerve in the neck include usually 2 cardiac nerves destined for the thorax.

Hypoglossal Nerve

As its name implies, the hypoglossal nerve, cranial nerve XII, innervates muscles of the tongue. Specifically, this nerve supplies the intrinsic muscles of the tongue and 3 extrinsic muscles that include the styloglossus, hyoglossus, and genioglossus. Primarily, these muscles retract, depress, and protrude the tongue, respectively.

Glossopharyngeal Nerve

Developmentally, the glossopharyngeal nerve, cranial nerve IX, is the cranial nerve of the third pharyngeal arch. In the neck, this nerve innervates the stylopharyngeus muscle and provides sensory innervation including taste to the posterior one-third of the tongue and supplies much of the pharyngeal mucosa. The typical complaint of a sore throat is mediated via the glossopharyngeal nerve. An additional branch travels to the carotid sinus and relays changes in blood pressure to the brainstem. Carotid sinus massage stimulates this branch with a resultant decrease in the heart rate/blood pressure.

Sympathetic Trunk

Generally, each spinal nerve of the body has an associated sympathetic ganglion. However, in the neck, these ganglia are usually combined to form superior, middle, and stellate ganglia. The superior ganglion is located just posterior to the internal carotid artery and connects with the upper 4 spinal nerves via 4 gray rami communicans, small branches that connect adjacent spinal nerves in the neck and carry postganglionic fibers. Cranially, the superior cervical ganglion has an extension known as the internal carotid nerve that travels with the internal carotid artery intracranially. An external carotid branch travels from the superior ganglion along the branches of the external carotid artery.

The middle and stellate ganglia connect to the fifth and sixth and seventh and eighth cervical spinal nerves, respectively. The middle cervical ganglion is located adjacent the cricoid cartilage at the sixth cervical vertebrae. The stellate ganglion is formed by the fusion of the inferior cervical and first thoracic ganglia and rests on the neck of the first rib just medial to the vertebral artery. Each cervical sympathetic ganglion issues a cardiac branch (postganglionic) that travels to the thorax for innervation of its viscera.

Accessory Nerve

After leaving the skull base, this nerve descends obliquely across the anterior surface of the transverse process of the atlas posterior to the digastric and stylohyoid muscles to enter the deep aspect of the superior part of the sternocleidomastoid muscle.

Vessels

Common Carotid Artery

The left and right common carotid arteries originate from the aorta and brachiocephalic artery, respectively. As these vessels ascend in the anterior triangle of the neck, they are enclosed with the laterally placed internal jugular vein and posteriorly placed vagus nerve in the carotid sheath. The common carotid arteries generally bifurcate into the laterally placed internal carotid and medially placed external carotid artery at the level of the C4 vertebrae or at the superior edge of the thyroid cartilage. At the proximal internal carotid artery, an enlargement is seen and is referred to as the carotid sinus. Pressure receptors are found in this structure. Near the carotid bifurcation, a chemoreceptor, the carotid body, is present.

The *internal carotid artery* travels on to enter the cranium and, therefore, does not supply structures in the neck. The *external carotid artery* supplies multiple branches to the exterior of the head and neck. Other arteries include:

- *Superior thyroid artery:* The first branch of the external carotid artery is the superior thyroid artery, which descends to the superior pole of the thyroid gland after first providing a superior laryngeal branch that enters the larynx via the thyrohyoid membrane.
- *Lingual artery:* The lingual artery, as its name implies, is destined to supply the tongue. This artery travels deep to the hyoglossus muscle.
- *Facial artery:* The facial artery extends from the external carotid artery, through or by the submandibular gland, over the mandible just anterior to the masseter muscle where its pulse is palpable, and terminates as the angular artery traveling toward the medial canthus of the orbit.
- *Ascending pharyngeal artery:* This vessel arises and travels superiorly toward the pharynx.
- *Occipital artery:* This vessel arises from the posterior aspect of the external carotid artery and travels to the scalp over the posterior head.
- *Posterior auricular artery:* This vessel also arises from the posterior external carotid artery and travels to the posterior scalp.

- *Maxillary artery:* This is 1 of the 2 terminal branches of the external carotid artery and soon after its origin travels deep to the neck of the mandible into the infratemporal fossa where it provides multiple branches that supply, for example, meningeal branches, branches to muscles of mastication and vessels to the maxillary sinus, the nasal cavity, and hard and soft palates.
- *Superficial temporal artery:* This artery and the maxillary are the 2 terminal branches of the external carotid artery. The superficial temporal artery travels cephalad through the parotid gland, anterior to the external auditory meatus, where its pulse can easily be palpated, and supplies the anterolateral scalp. Along its course, this vessel also provides branches to the face.

Internal Jugular Vein

The internal jugular vein is the primary venous outlet from the cranium and, as described earlier, travels in the anterior triangle of the neck within the carotid sheath. This vessel joins with the subclavian vein to form the brachiocephalic vein. Within the neck, main tributaries include pharyngeal branches, a common facial vein that receives the facial and lingual veins, and the superior and middle thyroid veins that drain the thyroid gland. The internal jugular vein can be cannulated for central venous access. A superficial landmark for this is to locate the interval between the sternal and clavicular heads of the sternocleidomastoid muscle.

Anterior Jugular Vein

This vessel, when present, travels on either side of the midline beginning just inferior to the chin and typically drains into the external jugular vein.

Subclavian Artery

As mentioned earlier, this vessel travels from the thorax through the superior thoracic aperture (i.e., root of the neck) and travels between the first rib and clavicle. While on the first rib, the subclavian artery is maintained between the anterior and middle scalene muscles. Three portions can therefore, be described. The first part is medial to the anterior scalene and gives rise to the vertebral artery, internal thoracic artery, and thyrocervical trunk. The second and most superior part is posterior to the anterior scalene and gives rise to the costocervical trunk. The third part of this vessel may give rise to the dorsal scapular artery if this does not arise from the transverse cervical artery (discussed later).

Vertebral Artery

The first branch of the subclavian artery is the vertebral artery. These vessels are important not only in supplying approximately one-third of the blood to the brain but also in supplying branches to the cervical spinal cord and adjacent muscles. This vessel begins by usually entering the transverse foramen of the sixth cervical vertebrae and then travels through the transverse foramina of the remaining cervical vertebrae to then enter the cranium.

Thyrocervical Trunk

This vessel is usually the second branch of the subclavian artery and generally provides 3 branches:

- *Inferior thyroid artery:* This is usually the first branch of the thyrocervical trunk and travels medially to supply the inferior pole of the thyroid and parathyroid glands. The terminal branches of the inferior thyroid artery are in intimate contact with the recurrent laryngeal nerve. An ascending cervical branch also extends from the inferior thyroid artery and travels parallel to the phrenic nerve on the anterior scalene muscle to supply muscular, vertebral, and spinal branches.
- *Transverse cervical artery:* This vessel travels through the posterior cervical triangle to the trapezius and rhomboid muscles.
- *Suprascapular artery:* This vessel also traverses the posterior triangle closer to the clavicle than the transverse cervical artery and terminates in the supra- and infraspinatus muscles.

Internal Thoracic Artery

This vessel arises usually just opposite to the origin of the thyrocervical trunk and descends into the thorax to supply anterior intercostals arteries and smaller branches to, for example, the thymus and sternum. Descriptions of its continuation will be discussed in the section on the thorax.

Costocervical Trunk

This branch of the second part of the subclavian artery divides into 2 branches:

- A descending branch known as the *highest intercostal artery* that supplies the first 2 posterior intercostals spaces and
- An ascending branch known as the *deep cervical artery* that ascends along the semispinalis cervicis muscle of the deep back muscles to form an anastomosis with a branch of the occipital artery

Dorsal Scapular Artery

If the transverse cervical artery does not give rise to a deep branch, then a dorsal scapular artery is usually found and will arise from the third part of the subclavian artery. This vessel then travels posteriorly to supply primarily the rhomboid muscles.

Lymphatics: Thoracic Duct

The thoracic duct is the primary lymphatic channel in the body and drains the entire body with the exception of the upper right half of the thorax, right upper limb, and right half of the head. This vessel begins in the abdomen and courses primarily in the thorax. Its termination is into the junction of the left subclavian vein and left internal jugular vein (venous angle); therefore, a portion of this structure is found in the left neck. In the neck, at approximately the seventh cervical vertebrae, the thoracic duct takes an outward curve between the carotid and vertebral arteries before emptying into the venous angle.

The major lymphatic vessels and nodes are found concentrated along the internal jugular vein and are referred to as the deep cervical chain. One of the larger of these is located in the angle created as the common facial vein drains into the internal jugular vein and is known as the *jugulodigastric node*. This node is a surgical landmark for identifying the common facial vein, which can be accessed for placing venous catheters into the internal jugular vein. Superficial nodes of the neck include submental, submandibular, anterior jugular, and external jugular groups.

Technique

THYROID LATERAL LOBE
COMMON CAROTID ARTERY
INTERNAL JUGULAR VEIN
Transverse
FIG. 9.1

Place the patient in a supine position with the neck extended over a small bolster and head turned to the side opposite the one being examined. Position the probe low in the neck with a transverse orientation. Navigate from midline-trachea and thyroid lateral lobes, then slide the probe laterally until the pulsating common carotid artery can be identified in contact with the lateral aspect of the thyroid lobe deep to sternocleidomastoid and infrahyoid muscles (e.g., omohyoid muscle, which "slips" between sternocleidomastoid and common carotid artery/internal jugular vein). The oval internal jugular vein (deforms/effaces with probe pressure) is typically immediately lateral to the common carotid artery. The internal jugular vein changes size (pulsates with respiratory

movement and noticeably enlarges with Valsalva and collapses on Valsalva release, and valves may be seen). Tilt/fan the probe to look for the vagus nerve in the groove between the posterior surfaces of the common carotid artery and internal jugular vein. Note the reflection and acoustic shadow of the cervical transverse process posterior to the common carotid artery and internal jugular vein (and longus colli). The anterolateral projection at the lateral extent of the transverse process is the anterior tubercle of the transverse process.

COMMON CAROTID ARTERY
CAROTID SINUS
INTERNAL CAROTID ARTERY
Longitudinal
FIG. 9.2

Place the patient in a supine position with the neck extended and head turned to the side opposite the one being examined. Starting from the previous image, center the probe over the common carotid artery and carefully rotate

Figure 9.1 Transverse view of the lateral lobe of the thyroid gland, common carotid artery, and internal jugular vein.

90 degrees clockwise to view the common carotid artery in its longitudinal axis. Slide the probe superiorly, keeping the common carotid artery in view until the expansion at the carotid sinus can be identified. Continue to slide the probe superiorly a short distance until the full extent of the carotid sinus can be seen (the superior, marker, end of the probe may need to be rotated slightly posteriorly while keeping the inferior heel of the probe stationary over the common carotid artery to identify, from inferior to superior, the common carotid artery, carotid sinus, and internal carotid artery).

INTERNAL CAROTID ARTERIES
EXTERNAL CAROTID ARTERIES
Transverse
FIG. 9.3

Place the patient in a supine position with the neck extended and head turned to the side opposite the one being examined. Center the probe over the carotid sinus and slowly rotate approximately 90 degrees counterclockwise. Then slide the probe superiorly until beyond the carotid bifurcation and both internal carotid artery and external carotid artery can be identified (in some patients, probe movement may be limited by contact against the angle of the mandible: patience and careful movement of the probe, patient head rotation, etc., will usually allow visualization of both the internal carotid artery and external carotid artery in transverse).

The internal carotid artery is larger than the external carotid artery and is located posterolaterally to the external carotid artery. The external carotid artery branches in the neck may be seen (superior thyroid artery) with careful observation and can also be distinguished based on flow dynamics (use of the spectral Doppler is beyond the scope of this text). The internal jugular vein is located lower in the neck (lateral to the external carotid artery, then lateral to the internal carotid artery), although in this image, the internal jugular vein has slipped between the internal carotid artery and the external carotid artery because of probe pressure. The internal jugular vein flattens/deforms/effaces with probe pressure, but arteries do not. Notice the transverse process with anterior and posterior tubercles and the hyperechoic honeycomb appearance of the vagus nerve.

COMMON CAROTID ARTERY
CAROTID SINUS
INTERNAL CAROTID ARTERY
EXTERNAL CAROTID ARTERY
Longitudinal
FIG. 9.4

From the preceding transverse image, determine the path an ultrasound (US) beam would have to follow to pass through both internal and external carotid arteries when the probe is rotated into the longitudinal axis (look at the previous image and draw an imaginary line from

Figure 9.2 Longitudinal view of common carotid artery, carotid sinus, and internal carotid artery.

the skin surface through sternocleidomastoid, internal carotid artery, and then external carotid artery). In this case the angle needed to image both vessels is fairly steep from posterolateral to anteromedial. The probe should be rotated into the longitudinal axis and the beam aimed along that imaginary line. Tilt/fan and adjust the probe's position until the common carotid artery, sinus, internal carotid artery, and external carotid artery can be seen within the image. Note that because the beam is traveling from posterolateral to anteromedial, the probe face is closest to internal carotid artery. As a result, the internal carotid artery appears in the near- to midfield of the image, and the external carotid artery, which is further from the probe face, appears deeper in the image (this mirror image orientation can be confusing early on). A similar image (mirror image in fact) could potentially be obtained by aiming the US beam along the same line but from anteromedial to posterolateral, although the contour of the neck and anterior edge of sternocleidomastoid might make that image more difficult to obtain. One or the other is inevitably easier to obtain based on the relative positions of external carotid artery/internal carotid artery in each patient.

VERTEBRAL ARTERY
Longitudinal
FIG. 9.5

Place the patient in a supine position and extend the neck, head turned away from the examination side, and begin with a longitudinal view of the common carotid artery (Figure 9.2), maintaining the same probe tilt and orientation. Slowly slide the probe face a short distance posteriorly along the neck, watching carefully for the reflections/acoustic shadows of cervical transverse processes to appear. Carefully adjust the probe tilt/angle/position until the anechoic vertebral artery can be seen between 2 transverse processes ("river under the bridge"). Keeping the vertebral artery segment in view, carefully slide the probe inferiorly until the artery can be seen "diving" toward the transverse foramen of CV6. In most patients, the vertebral artery can easily be followed further inferiorly to its origin from the

Figure 9.3 Transverse view of internal and external carotid arteries just superior to the bifurcation of common carotid artery.

subclavian artery. The vertebral vein may be seen anterior to the artery in the spaces between adjacent transverse foramina (acoustic shadows of transverse processes prevent US imaging of the vertebral vessels within the transverse foramina).

DEEP CERVICAL LYMPH NODE
Transverse
FIG. 9.6

Place the patient in a supine position with the neck extended over a small bolster. Orient the probe transversely with the common carotid artery and internal jugular vein in view (see Figure 9.1). Slowly slide the

probe superiorly, keeping the common carotid artery and internal jugular vein in view. Watch for the appearance of occasional small, ovoid, hypoechoic lymph nodes with a linear hyperechoic band/stripe in the center (fat tracking into the hilum along the afferent lymphatic vessel). Deep cervical nodes are seen at intervals along the anterior (medial), posterior (lateral), and superficial surfaces of internal jugular vein.

The US image shows the typical hypoechoic appearance of a lymph node with a hyperechoic stripe/band in the center (fat tracking into hilum along afferent lymph vessel), seen at the medial aspect of internal jugular vein.

Figure 9.4 Longitudinal (parasagittal oblique) view of common carotid artery, carotid sinus, internal carotid artery, and external carotid artery.

CLINICAL APPLICATIONS

For patients who are in hypovolemic shock or very ill, establishing a vascular access is one of the priorities after airway breathing is ensured. In cases in which peripheral venous access is not possible, central venous access is performed to allow fluid resuscitation, measurement of hemodynamics, and delivery of medications and nutritional support.

The most common access point for central venous catheterization is the internal jugular vein. Other veins can also be used, such as the femoral vein. US is used to identify the internal jugular vein through a supraclavicular approach visualizing the internal jugular vein at the lateral border of the clavicular head of the sternocleidomastoid. The vein can also be visualized between the 2 heads of the sternocleidomastoid muscle. The carotid arteries can be evaluated by color Doppler US for the detection of carotid artery stenosis and atherosclerotic plaques. Carotid US can accurately describe the location and internal characteristics, as well as the surface details of the carotid arteries. Specifically, the intima-media thickness is a measurable index for the degree of atherosclerosis in carotid arteries and is associated with increased risk factors for stroke. Similarly, the color Doppler can visualize the blood flow in the carotid vessels and identify stenotic segments. Specifically, when examining the vertebral artery, the flow direction is an important aspect in the diagnosis of proximal stenosis of the subclavian artery. The flow in the vertebral artery may be reversed in case of subclavian steal syndrome because of proximal stenosis of the subclavian artery.

Figure 9.5 Longitudinal view of the vertebral artery entering the transverse foramen of the sixth cervical vertebra and then between the sixth and fifth transverse foramina.

Figure 9.6 Transverse view of deep cervical lymph node, internal jugular vein, and common carotid artery.

Viscera of the Neck

Review of the Anatomy

The viscera of the neck include the submandibular gland, larynx, trachea, pharynx, esophagus, thyroid, and parathyroid glands.

Submandibular Gland

This second largest salivary gland is found overlying the posterior belly of the digastric and stylohyoid muscles. A smaller and deeper portion will also be found on the superior surface of the mylohyoid muscle. Sometimes, the gland connects with the parotid or sublingual gland through a glandular process. The duct of the submandibular gland (Wharton's duct) runs from its deep aspect or glandular hilum at the level of the mylohyoid muscle toward the medial aspect of the sublingual gland. The facial artery usually grooves or traverses the superficial portion of this gland on its way to the face. The lingual artery and vein run at its medial side. Autonomically, the submandibular gland receives its innervation via a branch of the facial nerve, cranial nerve VII.

Sublingual Gland

The sublingual gland is found at the floor of the mouth covered by the oral mucosa (small ducts open at the base of the sublingual fold) between the geniohyoid, intrinsic muscles of the tongue, hyoglossal muscle (medially), and the mylohyoid muscle. Its medial side is wrapped around the terminal part of the submandibular duct. It receives postganglionic parasympathetic fibers from the submandibular ganglion.

Larynx/Trachea

The larynx (voice box) is composed of 9 cartilages, 3 paired and 3 unpaired. The larger unpaired cartilages are the thyroid, cricoid, and epiglottis. The smaller paired cartilages are the arytenoids, corniculates, and cuneiforms. The epiglottis protects the inlet of the larynx, and the remaining cartilages provide support and, as related to the arytenoids, rotate and thereby cause tension or relaxation of the vocal cords. The recurrent laryngeal nerve innervates all muscles of the larynx with the exception of the cricothyroid muscle, which is innervated by the external laryngeal branch of the superior laryngeal nerve. The larynx terminates at the sixth cervical vertebrae and becomes the trachea, which continues inferiorly in the midline just anterior to the esophagus in the neck.

Pharynx/Esophagus

The pharynx, a thin, skeletal muscle semicylinder, begins at the base of the skull and descends to the sixth cervical vertebrae, where it becomes the narrowed esophagus. The pharynx is common to the air we breathe and the food we eat. It is composed of an inner mucosa, a pharyngobasilar fascia, and skeletal muscles that are divided into semicircular fibers known as the pharyngeal constrictors and longitudinal muscles such as the stylopharyngeus. The pharynx is coated posterolaterally by the buccopharyngeal fascia. This fascia is in intimate contact posteriorly with the prevertebral fascia. The fascial plane between these 2 fasciae extends inferiorly to the superior mediastinum; therefore, infections that penetrate the posterior wall of the pharynx can extend into the mediastinum and result in mediastinitis or endocarditis.

The pharynx is common to the nasal and oral cavities and larynx and collects and propels food toward the esophagus. The pharynx is innervated by the pharyngeal plexus whose primary motor input is via the vagus nerve. The sensory and sympathetic input to this plexus found primarily on the posterior aspect of the middle pharyngeal constrictor muscle is via the glossopharyngeal and cervical sympathetic trunk, respectively.

The pharynx is divided into a naso, oro, and laryngo (hypo) pharynx as it passes posterior to these regions. Important structures found in the nasopharynx include the pharyngeal tonsil and the medial opening of the Eustachian tube. The oropharynx contains the lingual and palatine tonsils, and the laryngopharynx houses the piriform recess, which is a common site for foreign objects (e.g., pills) to become entrapped.

Thyroid Gland

The thyroid gland contained in its own fibrous capsule is composed of left and right lateral lobes that are united across the midline by the isthmus that overlies the second through fourth tracheal rings. The thyroid gland regulates the rate of metabolism in the body by secreting thyroxine and thyrocalcitonin. It is covered superolaterally by the sternothyroid muscle and may have a cephalad extension called the pyramidal lobe, which is generally from the left lateral lobe. Remnants of the thyroglossal duct may also be found to extend from such a pyramidal lobe superiorly through the hyoid bone and even to the foramen cecum of the tongue. Cysts may develop along this duct and necessitate surgical removal. Its arterial supply is from the superior and inferior thyroid arteries, and its drainage is from the superior, middle, and inferior thyroid veins.

Parathyroid Glands

Normally located on the posterior aspect of the thyroid gland, the parathyroids are divided into 2 superior and 2 inferior glands. These structures maintain serum calcium levels and are derived from the fourth and third pharyngeal arches, respectively. The inferior parathyroids may sometimes be found in the thorax.

Technique

SUBMANDIBULAR SALIVARY GLAND
Longitudinal (Oblique Parasagittal)
FIG. 9.7

Place the patient in a supine position with the neck extended over a small bolster. Orient the probe approximately parallel to the inferior margin of the body of the mandible near the angle. Adjust the probe position until the fine-grained hyperechoic submandibular gland can be identified. Slide the probe medially and laterally and anteriorly and posteriorly to locate the gland in relationship to the posterior free edge of mylohyoid. The largest mass of the gland is superficial (inferior) to mylohyoid, but a small part of the gland conveying the submandibular duct curves up over the posterior free edge of mylohyoid to enter the oral cavity. In the US image shown, the gland was actively secreting and the anechoic fluid within the duct is clearly seen at the superior edge of mylohyoid surrounded by a small amount of glandular tissue.

SUBMANDIBULAR SALIVARY GLAND
Longitudinal (Oblique Coronal)
FIG. 9.8

Place the patient in a supine position with the neck extended over a small bolster. Orient the probe perpendicular to the inferior edge of the body of the mandible, with the marker side resting on the inferior edge of the mandible. The remainder of the probe should be faced against the skin of the neck and the beam aimed superiorly toward the oral cavity. Identify the fine-grained hyperechoic appearance of the submandibular gland and the reflection and acoustic shadow of the body of the mandible. Slide the probe anteriorly and posteriorly along the edge of the mandible, and identify the thin sheet of mylohyoid muscle at the gland's deep surface and the hypoechoic oval of intermediate tendon of digastric between mylohyoid and the deep surface of the gland. Look for pulsations of the facial artery deep to and

Submandibular gland

Mylohyoid m. posterior edge

Submandibular gland deep lobe with duct

Cerebellum

Brain

Top of head

Mylohyoid m. posterior edge

Submandibular gland

Submandibular gland deep lobe

Tongue

Submandibular duct

Figure 9.7 Longitudinal (oblique parasagittal) view of submandibular salivary gland and submandibular duct in relationship to the posterior free edge of mylohyoid muscle.

within the substance of the gland, usually near the posterior aspect of the gland. The tortuosity of the artery is seen as multiple sections of the artery in cross-section.

SUBLINGUAL SALIVARY GLANDS
Longitudinal (Coronal)
FIG. 9.9

Place the patient in a supine position with the neck extended over a small bolster. Orient the probe transversely (marker right) with the probe face against the skin of the neck just posterior to the inferior surface of the mental region of the mandible, with the beam aimed superiorly into the floor of the mouth. Identify from superficial (inferior) to deep (superior) the right and left anterior bellies of digastric (the reflections and acoustic shadows of the inferior margins of the mandibular bodies are just beyond the image edges on either side) and the thin sheet of the mylohyoid muscle, geniohyoid, and genioglossus muscles, with the right and left sublingual glands occupying the fatty spaces just lateral to geniohyoid/genioglossus. Tilt/fan the probe face to see the ovoid glands, which are slightly hypoechoic to the surrounding fat/connective tissue.

THYROID GLAND TRACHEA
Transverse
FIG. 9.10

Place the patient in a supine position with the neck extended over a small bolster. Place the probe transversely over skin of the neck few centimeters above the sternal notch. Adjust the probe's position until the lateral lobes of the thyroid gland (hyperechoic grainy appearance with multiple small anechoic vessels seen throughout) and the thin isthmus (anterior to the trachea) can be identified. The trachea appears hypoechoic

Figure 9.8 Longitudinal (oblique coronal) view of submandibular salivary gland, mandible, mylohyoid muscle, intermediate tendon of digastric muscle, and facial artery.

with a bright reflection anteriorly where the US beam leaves aqueous of thyroid mucosa and enters the tracheal air column (air-mucosa interface), and multiple thin hyperechoic bands are seen (reverberation artifact). Thin infrahyoid (strap) muscles are seen at the superficial surface of the thyroid isthmus and lateral lobes. The medial edges of sternocleidomastoid may be seen superficial to the infrahyoid muscles on either side of the image (only the right sternocleidomastoid is seen in this image). The esophagus is seen clearly in this image just to the left of the trachea (common position) at the posteromedial aspect of the left thyroid lobe. It typically has a bulls-eye appearance with concentric hypoechoic/hyperechoic rings. Ask the patient to swallow and see a hyperechoic "flash" of air artifact.

LATERAL THYROID LOBE
COMMON CAROTID ARTERY
INTERNAL JUGULAR VEIN
FIG. 9.11

Place the patient in a supine position with the neck extended over a small bolster. The probe slides laterally (from previous midline thyroid) until several structures can be identified: from medial to lateral, deep to sternocleidomastoid muscle (and in this location deep to omohyoid and sternohyoid muscles); lateral lobe of thyroid gland; common carotid artery; internal jugular vein; and anterior scalene muscle (from medial to lateral, useful landmarks for navigating, such as to scalene interval for brachial plexus). The omohyoid muscle (inferior belly) can be identified between the deep surface of sternocleidomastoid muscle and the internal jugular vein.

Figure 9.9 Longitudinal (coronal) view of sublingual salivary glands, anterior bellies of digastric, mylohyoid, geniohyoid, and genioglossus muscles.

CLINICAL APPLICATIONS

Salivary stones are most often located in the submandibular gland (60%-90% of cases) and may be multiple, causing **sialolithiasis**. Sialolithiasis can cause partial or total obstruction of the salivary duct. Salivary stones or sialoliths when present in the distal part of the submandibular duct (Wharton's duct) may be palpable in the floor of the mouth.

An autoimmune disease, **Sjögren syndrome** affects women over 40 years of age and is characterized by intense lymphocytic and plasma cell infiltration and destruction of salivary and lacrimal glands resulting in dry mouth and eyes. The most common malignant neoplasms occurring in salivary glands are mucoepidermoid carcinoma and adenoid cystic carcinoma.

Thyroid nodules are the most common finding on US examination (up to 50%). Approximately, 60% to 70% of these nodules are benign in nature and are benign follicular nodules or thyroiditis. Malignancy occurs in 5% to 7% of all thyroid nodules (papillary, follicular anaplastic, and medullary carcinomas); however, the lifetime risk of thyroid cancer is less than 1% in the United States.

Figure 9.10 Transverse view of thyroid gland lobes, thyroid isthmus, trachea, esophagus, and strap muscles.

Figure 9.11 Transverse view of right thyroid lobe, common carotid artery, internal jugular vein, vagus nerve, sternocleidomastoid, sternothyroid, omohyoid, and anterior scalene muscles.

Face

Review of the Anatomy

In general, the face is the region of the anterior head superiorly to the frontal bone, posteriorly to but not including the pinnae and inferiorly to the lower edge of the mandible. Not only are multiple organs of sense (eye, nasal, and oral cavities) located here but also the muscles that uniquely allow humans to communicate emotion (i.e., muscles of facial expression). Portions of glands (parotid, lacrimal) and muscles of mastication are also found on the face.

Fasciae/Connective Tissue

The face differs from the rest of the body in that its subcutaneous fat is completely separated from underlying muscles by investing fascia, which envelops the muscles. This superficial musculoaponeurotic system is a continuous, organized, fibrous network connecting the facial muscles with the dermis in the area of the forehead, parotid, zygomatic, infraorbital, nasolabial fold, and lower lip regions or the so-called facial ligaments. Additional defined fascial/connective tissue layers of the face include:

- **Galea aponeurotica:** this flattened tendon of the scalp connects the frontalis and occipitalis muscles and terminates on the zygomatic arch.
- **Deep cervical fascia:** continues cephalically to cover the parotid gland and masseter muscle.
  - *Parotid fascia:* splits into a deep and superficial layer to encapsulate the parotid gland. The deep layer forms a thickening known as the stylomandibular ligament that inserts onto the angle of the mandible. This ligament separates the parotid and submandibular glands. The parotid fascia extends cephalically to the zygomatic arch.
  - *Masseteric fascia:* continuous with the deeper layer of the temporal fascia and, specifically, its deeper lamina that attaches onto the lateral aspect of the zygomatic arch.

Muscles

Although some animals have muscles that move overlying skin, a human is unique in having a concentration of such muscles under the skin of the face. These muscles are used to convey facial expression/emotion and close/open the orifices (eye, nasal, and oral cavities) and are all innervated by the facial nerve. Some of the larger muscles of facial expression are found in Table 9.1. The last 2 muscles in the table (temporalis and masseter) are not muscles of facial expression but rather muscles of mastication that have a superficial position on the face. Therefore, they are not innervated by the facial nerve but by the mandibular division of the trigeminal nerve, which innervates all muscles of mastication.

Vessels

The major arterial blood vessels of the face are derived from the external carotid artery. Smaller branches of the internal carotid artery are also found on the face around the outer orbit. In general, same named veins travel with these external carotid branches. The following describe arterial branches:

- **Facial artery:** the facial artery extends from the external carotid artery, through or by the submandibular gland, over the mandible just anterior to the masseter muscle where its pulse is palpable, and terminates as the angular artery traveling toward the medial canthus of the orbit. After crossing the mandible, the facial artery provides several branches.
  - *Inferior labial:* supplies the lower lip
  - *Superior labial:* supplies the upper lip and nasal septum
  - *Lateral nasal:* supplies the ala and dorsum of the nose
  - *Angular:* supplies the orbicularis oculi and the lacrimal sac
- **Superficial temporal artery:** one of two terminal branches of the external carotid artery. Provides small branches to the parotid gland and anterior ear and then courses into the scalp as a terminal frontal and parietal branch. Larger branches before this termination include the following:
  - *Transverse facial branch:* travels superficial to the masseter superior to the zygomatic arch. Supplies the parotid gland and masseter muscle.
  - *Zygomaticoorbital branch:* travels to the lateral angle of the orbit and supplies the orbicularis oculi muscle.
- **Supraorbital artery:** a branch of the ophthalmic artery. On the face, it supplies regional muscles and anastomoses with the angular artery and frontal branch of the superficial temporal arteries.

TABLE 9.1   Large Muscles of Facial Expression

Muscle	Origin	Insertion	Action
Frontalis	Epicranial aponeurosis	Skin of eyebrows and root of the nose	Horizontally wrinkles the skin of the forehead (i.e., raises the eyebrows)
Corrugator supercilii	Medial superciliary arch	Skin over medial eyebrow	Vertically wrinkles the skin between the superciliary arches
Orbicularis oculi	Orbital rim	Skin overlying orbital rim, tarsal plates	Both parts (orbital/palpebral) close the eyelids
Procerus	Fascia of nasal bones and adjacent cartilages	Skin between superciliary arches	Horizontally wrinkles skin over the nasion
Nasalis	Maxillary bone	Ala of nose	Transverse portion constricts ala and alar portion widens the ala
Depressor septi nasi	Incisive fossa of maxillary bone	Ala and septum of nose	Widens nasal aperture
Levator labii superioris alaque nasi	Frontal process of maxillary bone	Skin of ala and upper lip	Elevates ala and upper lip
Levator labii superioris	Maxillary bone	Skin of upper lip	Elevates upper lip
Zygomaticus minor	Zygomatic bone	Upper lip	Elevates upper lip
Zygomaticus major	Zygomatic bone	Angle of mouth	Elevates upper lip
Orbicularis oris	Maxillary bone	Skin of lips	Closes mouth
Levator anguli oris	Maxillary bone	Angle of mouth	Elevates angle of mouth
Risorius	Masseteric fascia	Angle of mouth	Draws angle of mouth laterally
Depressor anguli oris	Oblique line of mandible	Angle of mouth	Depresses angle of mouth
Depressor labii inferioris	Oblique line of mandible	Skin of lower lip	
Mentalis	Incisive fossa of mandible	Skin of chin	Elevates and protrudes lower lip
Buccinator	Mandible, maxillary bone, and pterygomandibular raphe	Angle of mouth	Tenses skin over cheek and maintains food between occlusal surfaces of the molar teeth
Temporalis	Bones and fascia of the temporal fossa	Coronoid process and distally along anterior ramus to the retromolar triangle of mandible	Retracts and elevates mandible
Masseter	Zygomatic bone and its arch	Angle of mandible	Elevates

- **Supratrochlear artery:** a terminal branch of the ophthalmic artery. Supplies skin of the medial orbital region.
- **Dorsal nasal artery:** a terminal branch of the ophthalmic artery. Supplies the lacrimal sac and dorsum of the nose.
- **Lacrimal artery:** a branch of the ophthalmic artery. On the face, it supplies the lacrimal gland and upper eyelid.
  - *Zygomaticofacial artery:* a branch of the lacrimal artery that supplies skin over the cheek.
  - *Zygomaticotemporal artery:* a branch of the lacrimal artery that supplies skin over the temporal fossa (i.e., lateral forehead anterior to the hairline).
- **Infraorbital artery:** a branch of the maxillary artery that on the face supplies the skin and associated muscles in the infraorbital, lateral nasal, and superior labial regions.
- **Buccal artery:** a branch of the maxillary artery that supplies the buccinator muscles and the skin and mucous membrane of the cheek.
- **Mental artery:** a branch of inferior alveolar artery, which is a branch of the maxillary artery. It exits the mental foramen to supply adjacent skin and soft tissues.
- **Lymphatic vessels/nodes:** in general, lymphatic drainage from the conjunctiva, eyelids, central forehead, and lateral cheek pass to the anterior auricular and superficial and deep parotid nodes. Drainage from the external nose, cheeks, upper lip, and lateral parts of the lower lip drain directly into the submandibular lymph nodes. The central lower lip and chin drain into the submental nodes.
- **Facial vein**
  - *Deep facial branch:* this branch travels deeply and connects to the pterygoid venous plexus, which then has intracranial connections.
  - *Retromandibular:* this vessel is formed within the parotid gland at the posterior border of the ramus of the mandible by the maxillary and superficial temporal veins. Inferiorly, it has an anterior and posterior division. The anterior division contributes to the common facial vein as does the facial vein to then enter the internal jugular vein. The posterior division joins with the posterior auricular vein to form the external jugular vein.

Nerves

Cutaneous Nerves

The cutaneous nerves of the face are primarily derived from the trigeminal nerve and branches from all 3 of its divisions (ophthalmic, maxillary, and mandibular). These divisions are also abbreviated as V1, V2, and V3, respectively. A small area over the angle of the mandible is supplied by branches of the cervical plexus.

- **Ophthalmic nerve (V1)**
  - *Supraorbital nerve:* this branch supplies branches to the upper eyelid and then distributes to the skin of the forehead posteriorly to the vertex of the skull.
  - *Supratrochlear nerve:* this nerve provides branches to the upper eyelid and adjacent skin of the central forehead.
  - ***Infratrochlear nerve:*** supplies the skin of the eyelids and lateral nose.
  - *Lacrimal nerve:* after supplying the lacrimal gland, it is distributed to the upper eyelid.
  - *External nasal nerve:* an extension of the anterior ethmoidal nerve that supplies skin over the lower half of the nose.
- **Maxillary nerve (V2)**
  - *Infraorbital nerve:* supplies the lower eyelid, upper lip, and lateral nose.
  - *Zygomaticofacial nerve:* supplies skin over the prominence of the cheek.
  - *Zygomaticotemporal nerve:* supplies the anterior aspect of the temporal region (i.e., lateral region of the forehead).
- **Mandibular nerve (V3)**
  - *Mental nerve:* supplies the skin over the chin and lower lip.
  - *Buccal nerve:* supplies the skin overlying the buccinator muscle as well as the buccal gingival and adjacent mucosa.
  - *Auriculotemporal nerve* supplies the skin of the temporal region and also carries postganglionic parasympathetic "hitchhiking" fibers from the otic ganglion that leave the auriculotemporal nerve and travel to the parotid gland. Fibers are also found traveling to the anterior pinnae and the temporomandibular joint.
- **Great auricular nerve:** derived from fibers of C2 and C3 from the cervical plexus and is primarily distributed to the skin over the parotid gland and ear lobe. In addition, some fibers supply the skin over the angle of the mandible.

Motor Nerves

Classically, all but 2 muscles of the face receive their innervation via the facial nerve, although the trigeminal nerve innervates the temporalis and masseter muscles found superficially on the face.

- **Facial nerve:** At the skull base, the facial nerve leaves the stylomastoid foramen and travels medially toward the face. This nerve travels through the parotid gland and forms an upper **temporofacial** and lower **cervicofacial** division. Five branches emanate from these divisions and will supply the muscles of facial expression. These branches coalesce as they approach the muscles of facial expression forming the so-called **pes anserine**.

- *Temporal branches:* innervate the frontalis, orbicularis oculi, and corrugator supercilii muscles.
- *Zygomatic branches:* innervate the orbicularis oculi and zygomaticus major muscles.
- *Buccal branches:* innervate the procerus, levator labii superioris alaeque nasi, levator labii superioris, levator anguli oris, zygomaticus minor (when present), zygomaticus major, buccinator, risorius, levator anguli oris, orbicularis oris, nasalis, and depressor anguli oris.
- *Marginal mandibular branches:* cross superficial to the facial vessels over the mandible and innervate the depressor anguli oris, depressor labii inferioris, mentalis, and orbicularis oris.
- *Cervical branch:* innervates the platysma muscle.
- **Trigeminal nerve: mandibular nerve (V3)**
  - *Masseteric nerve:* supplies the masseter muscle and temporomandibular joint.
  - *Deep temporal nerves:* Two to three in number supply the overlying temporalis muscle.
- **Sympathetics**
  - *External carotid plexus:* These postganglionic sympathetic fibers derived from the superior cervical ganglion of the sympathetic trunk within the neck travel along branches of the external carotid artery that are destined for the face (e.g., facial and superficial temporal arteries). These fibers are vasoconstrictive, secretory, and pilomotor in nature.

Viscera

The viscera of the face include the parotid and lacrimal glands, external aspect of the eyeball, and opening to the oral cavity.

- **Parotid gland:** This is the largest of the salivary glands and is situated anterior to the ear and inferior to the zygomatic arch and dips inferior to the level of the mandible at the retromandibular fossa. It is invested with a dense fibrous capsule, the parotid sheath. The course of the facial nerve through the parotid gland artificially divides the parotid gland into superficial and deep parts. This gland receives its innervation from postganglionic fibers derived from the glossopharyngeal nerve (ninth cranial nerve) that have synapsed in the otic ganglion and then have traveled along the auriculotemporal nerve, which is a branch of the mandibular division (V3) of the trigeminal nerve. The parotid gland contains a parotid duct (Stensen's duct) that travels inferior to the zygomatic arch and then empties into the vestibule of the mouth, between the cheek and the upper second molar tooth. An accessory parotid gland (socia parotidis) may be seen extending medially along the parotid duct, which enters the oral cavity adjacent to the upper second molar tooth after piercing the buccinator muscle. Regionally, the buccal fat pad is seen and separates the masseter from the buccinator muscles. Loss of or absence of this pad results in dimpling of the skin of the cheek.
- **Lacrimal gland:** This is the tear-secreting gland of the body located in the superolateral aspect of the orbit. The superficial aspect of this gland is seen from the facial perspective. The superficial and deep portions of the lacrimal gland are separated by the tendon of the levator palpebrae superioris muscle. Innervation to the lacrimal gland is derived from the facial nerve. Postganglionic fibers leave the pterygopalatine ganglion and travel with branches of the maxillary and ophthalmic divisions of the trigeminal nerve to terminate onto the lacrimal gland.
- **Eye:** The external aspect of the eyeball is seen on the face as the cornea, sclera, and overlying bulbar conjunctiva.
- **Lips:** These extensions of the oral cavity are composed primarily of skin, muscles, mucosa, interposed vessels and nerves, and minor salivary glands. The **vermillion border** is the demarcation between the reddened vascular edge of the lips and adjacent skin.

Technique

**PAROTID GLAND
SALIVARY GLAND**
Transverse
FIG. 9.12

Place the patient in a supine position with the neck extended over a small bolster. Turn the head of the patient to the side opposite the one being examined. Orient the probe transversely under the ear lobe. Place the anterior edge of the probe over the mandible (acoustic shadow), masseter (typical hypoechoic muscle appearance with hyperechoic connective tissue bands), and the posterior edge over the sternocleidomastoid muscle. Tilt/fan the probe for the best image of parotid gland tissue that appears as fine grain slightly hyperechoic. Because the parotid gland tends to attenuate US energy, it is often not possible to observe its deep surface. However, the external carotid artery and the retromandibular vein can often be seen at the deep aspect of the parotid gland.

CLINICAL APPLICATIONS

US imaging of the parotid gland is mainly performed when there is a parotid gland swelling. Inflammatory diseases are the most common diseases affecting the salivary glands. In acute inflammation, salivary glands are enlarged and hypoechoic. Viral salivary gland infections are the most common in children. **Parotitis** is a viral infection (mumps) of the parotid gland, which results in glandular swelling. Glandular swelling stretches the capsule and the fascia of the parotid gland resulting in considerable pain.

Benign neoplasms such as **pleomorphic adenomas** (mixed tumor) and Warthin tumors (adenolymphoma, cystadenolymphoma, papillary cystadenoma lymphomatosum) are slowly growing, painless masses of the parotid gland. The most common malignant neoplasms occurring are mucoepidermoid carcinoma and adenoid cystic carcinoma. Salivary glands may also be affected by lymphoma as a painless, progressive swelling. They are usually associated with autoimmune disease, most often Sjögren syndrome. HIV-positive patients often have sialolithiasis and swelling of the parotid glands.

Figure 9.12 Transverse view of parotid salivary gland, masseter, and mandible.

Eye and Orbit

Review of the Anatomy

The eyeball (globe) is located anteriorly in the bony orbit, covered anteriorly by the eyelids. Most of the remainder of the orbit is occupied by orbital fat. The numerous nerves and vessels serving the eye, eyelids, and face around the orbit, plus the extraocular muscles that move the eye, all traverse the orbital fat to reach the eye or other targets within and around the orbit.

The deep surfaces of the eyelids are covered by **conjunctiva**, which then reflects over the **sclera** (the white outer layer of the eye) and attaches along the corneoscleral junction. The conjunctiva forms a sac when the eyelids are closed, which contains a thin layer of lacrimal gland secretions.

The wall of the eyeball consists of 3 layers. The outer fibrous layer is made up mainly by the sclera, plus the (normally) transparent cornea anteriorly. The middle vascular layer consists of the choroid posteriorly, which is continuous with the ciliary body and iris anteriorly. The ciliary body, which extends anteriorly from the choroid, is a circumferential triangular elevation consisting of ciliary muscles, ciliary processes, and ciliary epithelium. The pigmented iris extends anteriorly from the ciliary body over the anterior surface of the lens with a central opening, the pupil. The inner layer consists of the visual (neural) retina posteriorly and the nonvisual retina anteriorly. The choroid layer is attached to the retina internally and the sclera externally.

The **lens**, a normally transparent biconvex disc, is suspended behind the iris via a circumferential system of zonular fibers attached to the lens capsule centrally and projections (ciliary processes) from the ciliary body peripherally. Collectively, the zonular fibers make up the suspensory ligament of the lens.

The interior of the eye is described as containing 3 chambers: the anterior chamber, the posterior chamber, and the vitreous chamber. The anterior chamber is located between the posterior (inner) surface of the cornea anteriorly and the anterior surfaces of the iris and lens posteriorly. The small posterior chamber is located between the posterior surface of the iris and the anterior surface of the lens. The anterior and posterior chambers contain aqueous humor. **Aqueous humor** is secreted from the ciliary epithelium into the posterior chamber and flows into the anterior chamber through the pupil. The vitreous chamber, occupied by the gelatinous vitreous humor, is located in the remainder of the globe between the posterior surface of the lens anteriorly and the retina posteriorly.

The central processes of retinal ganglion cells converge at the optic disc to form the optic nerve (CN II), which exits the posteromedial aspect of the eye and traverses the orbital fat to exit the orbit posteriorly via the optic canal. The optic nerve is surrounded by a sheath consisting of all 3 meningeal layers: dura, subarachnoid, and pia. The subarachnoid space of the optic nerve sheath is continuous with the intracranial subarachnoid space.

Technique

EYE AND OPTIC NERVE
Transverse
FIG. 9.13

A high-resolution linear array US transducer should be selected for examination of the eye and optic nerve. The patient should be in a supine position and the examination is performed with the eyes closed. A generous amount of standard water-soluble US gel should be applied to the closed eyelids so that the probe face stands off from contact with the eyelids and very minimal pressure is applied to the eye through the probe face. In some patients, the use of sterile US gel may be indicated (the presence of cuts or lacerations of the eyelids for example) and additionally, a sterile occlusive dressing can be placed over the closed eyelids before applying gel.

The patient's eyes should be closed. Ask the patient to look straight ahead. Place the probe transversely over the eyelids/eye with the probe marker side directed to the right. Adjust the scan depth so that the entire globe and anterior 1 to 1.5 cm of orbital fat behind the globe are visible in the image. Carefully adjust the probe position and tilt as needed (remind the patient to look straight ahead) to identify, from anterior to posterior, the eyelid, the thin anechoic stripe of fluid in the conjunctival sac, the hyperechoic curving surface of the cornea parallel to the eyelid, the iris and pupil, the hyperechoic anterior and posterior reflections of the lens capsule (along with the normally anechoic lens between), and the ciliary body extending posteriorly from the iris. Identify the anechoic aqueous humor within the anterior and posterior chambers and the anechoic vitreous humor within the vitreous chamber. The retinal and choroid layers cannot be resolved separately with US examination, appearing as a thin hypoechoic stripe lining the interior of the globe just outside the vitreous chamber (there is often a hyperechoic line at the inner surface of the retina where it is perpendicular to the US beam). Adjust the probe position and tilt as needed until the hypoechoic optic nerve can be seen exiting the globe posteriorly.

CLINICAL APPLICATIONS

US examination of the eye is commonly used in emergency departments for examination of structures of the eye in patients with traumatic injuries involving the orbit/eye. US examination is contraindicated when rupture of the globe is clinically suspected, as any pressure applied to the ruptured eye can result in further extrusion of eye contents/humors.

US can be used to examine the eye when direct examination and funduscopy are not possible because of eyelid edema or hematoma or hemorrhage in the anterior chamber (hyphema). US examination of the eye can be used to detect globe wall perforation, intraocular foreign bodies, lens dislocation/subluxation, cataracts, vitreous hemorrhage, retinal detachment, hyaloid/vitreous detachment, and choroidal detachment. There are also US techniques for testing the pupillary light reflex when the pupil cannot be directly examined.

US measurement of the optic nerve/optic nerve sheath diameter is used when elevated intracranial pressure is suspected, such as in patients with head injuries, altered consciousness, or possible intracranial hemorrhage. Swelling/enlargement of the optic nerve and its sheath has been shown to develop earlier in the course of elevated intracranial pressure than swelling of the optic disc/papilledema. US examination is also used in the evaluation of posterior wall (retinal/choroidal) or optic nerve sheath masses such as primary benign or malignant tumors or metastases.

Labels in figure: Fluid in conjunctival sac, Eyelid, Cornea, Anterior chamber, Iris, Pupil, Ciliary body, Lens, Posterior chamber, Optic disc, Vitreous chamber, Retina / choroid, Orbital fat, Optic n. & sheath

Figure 9.13 Transverse view of orbital contents, including the eye, optic nerve, and orbital fat. Transverse section of cadaveric orbit/eye from NIH Visible Human Project.

10

Female Pelvis

Review of the Anatomy

The general anatomical presentation of the pelvis is described in Chapter 11. This chapter focuses specifically on the elements of the female pelvis. However, there are some differences noted when comparing the pelvises of males and females. In females, the pelvis is typically smaller in size, denser, and less thick than in males. In comparison, the female pelvic cavity has less depth and width, the **pubic arch** (also known as the subpubic angle) is greater in size, and the greater sciatic notch is broader. When detailing the pelvic inlet, the males have a heart-shaped appearance, whereas the female pelvis is described as having an oval-shaped inlet. The pelvic outlet, on the other hand, is also bigger in females as a result of the outward protuberance of the ischial tuberosities. Lastly, the obturator foramen is described as being triangular or egg-shaped in females compared with a more rounded shape found in males.

In females, the **ureter**s and the ovarian vessels are found traveling together along the pelvic brim (linea terminalis) and are crossed superficially by the uterine arteries. As a result of this anatomical arrangement, there is a potential risk of injury to the ureters when performing an oophorectomy or hysterectomy. In males, the ureters enter the bladder at the posterolateral surface by coursing behind and inferiorly to the ductus deferens and anteriorly to the seminal vesicles. In females, the urethra is short in length, roughly 4 cm, and is observed passing through the pelvic floor into the perineum and opening into the vestibule of the vagina.

Uterus

The uterus is a muscular organ and the largest female reproductive organ. It is supported and kept in place by numerous ligaments such as the round, broad, and cardinal ligaments, as well as the rectouterine, pubocervical, and uterosacral ligaments (described as follows). In females, the uterus occupies the space between the bladder and rectum at the level of the pelvic midline. The uterus allows for implantation of the fertilized oocyte and sustains life for the developing fetus until delivery. The main arterial source is the uterine artery, with contributions from the ovarian artery.

The uterus is anatomically grouped into a cervix, isthmus, body, and fundus. The cervix is located at the most inferior portion of the uterus and serves as a connection between the vagina and the uterus. The isthmus is a tapered (approximately 1 cm) portion of the uterus between the body and the cervix. The body, which is the largest segment of the uterus, contains the uterine cavity. The fundus is a rounded structure located at the upper region of the uterus. The uterine cavity joins with the cervical canal, which opens into the vaginal canal. The normal position of the uterus is **anteverted** (the cervical canal is turned anteriorly at approximately right angles to the vaginal canal) and **anteflexed** (the uterine cavity is bent slightly forward relative to the cervical canal). When the urinary bladder is filled, it displaces the uterus posteriorly, opening the angle between the vaginal and cervical canals.

Ligaments

There are various prominent peritoneal ridges or ligaments found within the pelvis of females, including the broad ligament of the uterus; round ligament of the uterus; ovarian ligament; suspensory ligament of the ovary; lateral, cardinal, or transverse cervical ligament; pubocervical ligament; pubovesical ligament; and uterosacral ligament.

The broad ligament of the uterus originates at the lateral border of the uterus and reaches the lateral pelvic wall. It comprises 2 layers of peritoneum and functions to hold the uterus in position. Many structures are found within the ligament, including the uterine tube, vessels, round ligament of the uterus, ovarian ligament, uterovaginal nerve plexus, lymphatics, and lower ureter. The broad ligament is subdivided into the mesovarium, mesosalpinx, and mesometrium. The mesovarium extends from in front of the ovary to the posterior border of the broad ligament; it is important to note that the mesovarium does not contain the ovary. The mesosalpinx aids in suspending the fallopian (uterine) tube. The mesometrium is inferior to the mesosalpinx and mesovarium and is a major contributor to the broad ligament.

The round ligament of the uterus runs within the (anterior/superior) layer of the broad ligament. It serves to hold the uterus anteverted and anteflexed by supporting the fundus of the uterus forward. The ligament attaches to the uterus anteriorly below the fallopian tubes. The round ligament passes through the inguinal canal at the deep inguinal ring and exits at the superficial inguinal ring. The ovarian ligament and suspensory ligament both attach to the ovary. The ovarian ligament is found below the uterine tubes and attaches from the ovary to the uterus. It consists of a fibromuscular cord coursing within the broad ligament. The suspensory ligament of the ovary, on the other hand, is a band of peritoneum, which attaches the ovary to the pelvic wall. It carries the ovarian vessels, nerves, and lymphatics.

The cardinal ligament (of Mackenrodt) extends from the cervix and vagina to the pelvic walls, traveling inferior to the base of the broad ligament. The cardinal ligament is composed of fibromuscular pelvic fascia and functions to provide support to the uterus.

The pubocervical ligament is composed of bands of connective tissue and connects the posterior border of the pubis to the cervix of the uterus. The pubovesical ligament travels from the neck of the bladder to the pelvic bone, whereas the uterosacral ligament, a firm fibromuscular band of pelvic fascia, attaches to the lower portion of the sacrum and extends to the cervix and the upper portion of the vagina.

The rectouterine ligament maintains the anatomical position of the cervix upwards and posteriorly. Occasionally, the rectouterine ligament may create a fold of peritoneum, known as the rectouterine fold. This fold extends across the isthmus of the uterus and attaches laterally to the rectum at the posterior wall of the pelvis.

At the pelvic inlet, the inferior portions of the abdominal peritoneum drapes over the pelvic viscera. In females, the abdominal peritoneum covers the fundus and body of the uterus and extends laterally over the uterine tubes to the pelvic walls, forming the broad ligament of the uterus. Peritoneum spanning the anterior/inferior aspect of the uterus reflects onto the urinary bladder forming a relatively shallow space called the vesicouterine pouch. The peritoneum covering the posterior/superior aspect of the uterus and uterine cervix descends to the superior border of the posterior vaginal fornix and then reflects onto the anterior surface of the rectum, forming a deep potential space known as the rectouterine pouch (of Douglas). The rectouterine pouch is the deepest peritoneal space in the supine position.

Ovaries

The ovaries are the female reproductive organs covered by germinal epithelial, which is closely related to embryologic peritoneum. The ovaries are not invested within the broad uterine ligament. Each ovary is suspended by **mesovarium**, which attaches the ovaries to the posterior/superior layer of the broad ligament. The suspensory (infundibulopelvic) ligament is anchored at the pelvis side wall and connects to the ovaries and thus also maintains the position of the ovaries along with the mesovarium. The ovarian ligament attaches the ovaries to the uterus. The ovaries are bordered by the external and internal iliac vessels on the lateral walls of the pelvis. The ovarian arteries are the main arterial supply to the ovaries and also form an anastomosis with the uterine artery. The ovarian arteries can be found within the suspensory (infundibulopelvic) ligament. Venous blood from the ovaries is collected by the left and right ovarian veins; the right ovarian vein drains into the inferior vena cava, whereas the left ovarian vein drains into the left renal vein.

Uterine Tubes (Fallopian Tubes)

The uterine tubes project laterally from the junction of the fundus and body of the uterus and open into the peritoneal cavity adjacent to the ovaries. The uterine tubes have fringelike appendages called fimbriae at the termination near the ovaries. The uterine tubes can be divided into 4 parts: infundibulum, ampulla, isthmus, and uterine part. An oocyte is expelled into the abdominal cavity from the ovaries during ovulation and is transferred to the uterus via the uterine tubes. The transport of oocytes is due to sweeping motions of the uterine tube fimbriae, the muscular contraction of the uterine tubes, and the ciliary motions of cilia lining the inner epithelial cells of the uterine tubes.

Vagina

The vaginal canal extends inferiorly from the cervix and terminates at the vaginal vestibule in the perineum. It serves to excrete menstrual products and receives the penis and ejaculate during intercourse. The vestibule is partially surrounded by the hymen, which is a membranous fold that degenerates after first coitus. The vagina receives its blood supply from the vaginal branches of the uterine and internal iliac arteries. It is supported in the pelvis by the levator ani, the urogenital diaphragm, and the perineal body. The nerves innervating the upper three-fourths of the vagina comes from the uterovaginal plexus, whereas the lower one-fourth is innervated by the deep perineal branch of the pudendal nerve. Internal iliac nodes drain lymphatics from the upper three-fourths of the vagina, whereas the superficial inguinal nodes drain lymphatics from the lower one-fourth portion of the vagina.

Technique

Transabdominal (Suprapubic) Views of Abdomen/Pelvis

SUPRAPUBIC FEMALE PELVIS
Longitudinal (Sagittal/ Parasagittal)
FIG. 10.1

This examination is best done when the patient's urinary bladder is full. If the urinary bladder is not at least partially full, bowel gas shadowing can interfere substantially with ultrasound (US) examination in this area. A full bladder displaces loops of bowel superiorly and provides an excellent acoustic window for US examination of pelvic structures behind the bladder.

With the patient in the supine position and properly draped, the heel of a curved array probe (nonmarker side) should be placed just over (or just above) the pubic symphysis with the marker side directed toward the head. Adjust the probe position and tilt until pelvic landmarks and structures can be identified. Urine, like all fluids, appears anechoic, and the bladder wall appears hyperechoic. In longitudinal views, full bladders are roughly triangular in shape with the apex pointing superiorly.

Posterior to the bladder, identify the **fundus** and body of the uterus, the hyperechoic endometrial stripe, and the cervix. The **myometrium** typically has a hypoechoic speckled appearance. Note the shape and position of the uterus, which changes with bladder filling. The endometrium appears as a hyperechoic stripe, which varies in thickness with the phase of the menstrual cycle. A thin hyperechoic vaginal stripe can often be identified extending inferiorly from the uterine cervix posterior to the bladder.

Identify the locations of the potential spaces, the rectouterine and vesicouterine pouches.

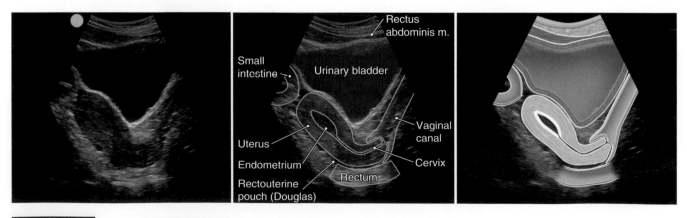

Figure 10.1 Normal longitudinal (sagittal/parasagittal) suprapubic view of the female pelvis.

After completing the suprapubic examination of the pelvis in the longitudinal plane, rotate the probe 90 degrees counterclockwise so that the marker side is directed to the right and position the probe face just superior to the pubic symphysis. Adjust the probe position and tilt until pelvic landmarks and structures can be identified. In transverse views, full bladders are roughly rectangular in shape.

Identify the **bladder**, uterus, and **endometrial stripe.** Scan carefully superiorly and inferiorly along the uterus and uterine cervix. Attempt to identify the right and left ovaries, which are commonly found alongside the body of the uterus and posterior/inferior to the external iliac vessels. Ovaries are often described as having a "chocolate-chip cookie" US appearance, where the "chips" are anechoic/hypoechoic ovarian follicles and the "cookie" is the more echogenic ovarian stroma.

Figure 10.2 Normal transverse suprapubic view of the female pelvis.

CLINICAL APPLICATIONS

Focused Assessment with Sonography for Trauma (FAST) Examination for Detection of Intraperitoneal Bleeding

In the supine patient, free intraperitoneal fluid or large amounts of blood from the abdominal viscera typically accumulate in the following locations: hepatorenal space (Morison's pouch), splenorenal space, and pelvis, in the pouch of Douglas in females and the retrovesical pouch in males. Chapter 12 describes the FAST examination performed to identify these spaces with examples of fluid accumulation.

Ectopic Pregnancy

Ectopic pregnancy is defined as the pregnancy in which the embryo is implanted outside the normal intrauterine location. This accounts for approximately 2% of all pregnancies in the United States, which increases to 18% in patients with first-trimester bleeding. The most common ectopic locations include the fallopian tube, abdomen, ovary, uterine interstitium, prior surgical scar, and cervix. Approximately 95% of all ectopic pregnancies take place within the uterine tubes. A US examination will show an extraovarian adnexal mass and an empty uterus.

Fibromyoma (Leiomyoma)

Fibromyomas or **leiomyomas** are the most common benign tumors of the uterus. These are primarily composed of smooth muscle and connective tissue. They are the most common cause of dysmenorrhea, pain, bleeding, and heavy menstrual cycles. They are commonly identified by use of US and surgically removed.

Endometriosis and Endometrial Cancer

Endometriosis is a mass of endometrial tissue such as stroma and glands that appears as a cyst and occurs in different extraendometrial locations such as uterine walls and ovaries. The majority of the adnexal masses, however, are benign masses.

The most common type of uterine cancer in approximately 90% of the cases is an **endometrial cancer**. It develops from the endometrium of the uterus. The symptoms are similar to endometriosis, such as vaginal bleeding, pain, and pelvic cramping. A US examination can detect both endometriosis and endometrial cancer. In contrast, ovarian tumors are typically assessed with endovaginal ultrasonography with color Doppler specifically identifying vascularized tissue, thick septations, and solid parts of the tumor.

11

Male Pelvis

Review of the Anatomy

The pelvis (Latin for "basin") is a bowl-shaped bony structure positioned superior to the lower limbs and inferior to the abdomen. The bones of the pelvis are the **os coxae** (2 hip bones), **sacrum**, and **coccyx**. The pelvis is divided by the linear terminalis (pelvic brim) into the lesser above and the greater pelvis below. The pelvic outlet is situated in the lesser pelvis and is sealed by the musculature of the pelvic floor, the coccygeus and the levator ani. The pelvis sits in an angled position, with the vertical axis in line with the anterior superior iliac spine and pubic tubercles, and the horizontal axis containing the coccyx and upper margin of the pubic symphysis. Thus, the pelvic cavity is parallel to the curvature of the sacrum.

The pelvis is also subdivided into an inlet and an outlet portion. The pelvic inlet, also known as the upper pelvic aperture, is the upper border of the pelvic cavity and is made up of 3 main parts, the sacral, iliac, and pubic portions. It has an almost entirely bony margin (linea terminalis) along the sacral promontory, ala of sacrum, arcuate line, pectineal line, pubic crest, and pubic symphysis. The sacrum, along with the anterior border of the ala of sacrum, makes up the sacral portion, forming the posterior border of the pelvic inlet. The iliac portion corresponds to the lateral border of the pelvic inlet, which is confined by the arcuate or iliopectineal line of the ilium. Finally, the pubic portion of the pelvic inlet is the upper border and includes the superior margin of the public symphysis. The pelvic inlet is mostly narrow and heart-shaped in males. At the pelvic inlet, the pelvic viscera is covered by the inferior aspect of the abdominal peritoneum. In males, peritoneum covering the urinary bladder reflects onto the anterior surface of the rectum, giving rise to the rectovesical pouch, a pocket that contains peritoneal fluid and some parts of the small intestine. The rectovesical pouch is also the most dependent area of the peritoneal cavity when positioned in a supine orientation.

The pelvic outlet is a diamond-shaped aperture that leads into the perineum. It has bony (ischiopubic rami) and ligamentous (sacrotuberous) margins secured in position by the pelvic and urogenital diaphragms. Specifically, the pelvic outlet is confined laterally by the ischial tuberosities and sacrotuberous ligaments, posteriorly by the sacrum and coccyx, and anteriorly by the pubic symphysis, arcuate pubic ligament, and rami of the pubis and ischium.

The musculature of the pelvic floor, known as the **pelvic diaphragm**, is composed mainly of the right and left levator ani muscles and completed posteriorly by the coccygeus muscles and their perineal fascia. The pelvic diaphragm acts to support all the pelvic viscera, flexes the anorectal junction during excretion, and helps in voluntary micturition (urination).

The pelvic walls are made up of bone (os coxae and sacrum), ligaments (sacrospinous and sacrotuberous), and muscles (obturator internus and piriformis). There are foramina in the pelvic walls, the greater and lesser sciatic foramina posteriorly and the obturator foramen anteriorly. The majority of the obturator foramen is enclosed by the obturator membrane, but a small obturator canal remains open anterosuperiorly.

The joints of the pelvis include the lumbosacral, sacroiliac, sacrococcygeal joints and the pubic symphysis. The lumbosacral joint is located between the L5 vertebra and base of the sacrum. The joint is accompanied by the intervertebral disc and bolstered by the iliolumbar ligaments. The sacroiliac joint is situated between the articular surfaces of the sacrum and ilium. It is a combined synovial and cartilaginous joint, surrounded by cartilage and held by the anterior, posterior, and interosseous sacroiliac ligaments. The sacrococcygeal joint is positioned between the sacrum and coccyx. It is a cartilaginous joint that is reinforced with the anterior, posterior, and lateral sacrococcygeal ligaments. Finally, the pubic symphysis, a cartilaginous or fibrocartilaginous joint, is found between the pubic bones in the median plane.

In males, the pelvic ligaments observed include the puboprostatic ligament, which is a condensation of the pelvic fascia and attaches from the prostate gland and continues to the pelvic bone. The inferior pubic or arcuate pubic ligament is found in both males and females. This ligament stretches across the inferior aspect of the pubic symphysis to connect with the medial surface of the inferior pubic rami.

Ureters and Urinary Bladder

The **ureters** are muscular conduits for urine extending from the kidneys to the urinary bladder. The ureters are made of smooth muscles and transitional epithelium and propel urine via peristaltic waves. The ureters cross the pelvic brim superior to the common iliac artery bifurcation after which they descend laterally into the pelvic wall. The ureters travel medial to the umbilical artery and the obturator vessels and posteroinferiorly to the ductus deferens and anterior to the seminal vesicles before flowing into the posterolateral surface of the bladder. Through its course, there are 3 points of constriction—at the ureteropelvic junction, when it travels across the pelvic brim; at the point where it crosses the common iliac artery; and at its entrance into the bladder.

The ureters enter the bladder at the base on a slant. They possess a slitlike orifice that functions as a valve, whereas the intramural portion of the ureters has circular fibers operating as a sphincter. Thus, when the bladder becomes distended, the valve and sphincter work to prevent the reflux of urine back into the ureters.

The **urinary bladder** is situated in the midline of the pelvis anteriorly, and the rectum occupies the midline of the pelvis posteriorly. It is made up of bundles of smooth muscles known as the detrusor muscle and is located inferior to the peritoneum. As the bladder fills, it extends toward the pelvic brim. Anatomically, the apex of the bladder is located anteriorly, and the fundus of the bladder forms the posteroinferior triangular aspect. At the urinary bladder's fundus there is a triangular section (bladder trigone) where the bladder mucosa is tightly bound to the underlying smooth muscle layer that lines the base of the bladder. The bladder trigone is surrounded by 2 openings of the ureters and the internal urethral orifice that has the internal sphincter. The neck of the bladder, which is at the fundus, leads into the urethra. The arterial blood supply for the bladder comes from the superior and inferior vesical arteries. The vesical plexus (or prostatic) drains the venous blood toward the internal iliac vein. The vesical and prostatic nervous plexuses innervate the bladder. The parasympathetic pelvic splanchnic nerves (S2–S4) function to contract the bladder and the detrusor muscle and also relax the internal urethral sphincter to initiate emptying of the bladder. The sympathetic nerves relax the bladder walls and constrict the internal urethral sphincter.

The urinary bladder empties into the urethra, which propels the urine to the exterior. In males, the urethra also functions for the passage of semen. The urethra passes through the prostate, the deep perineal pouch (membranous part), and the penis (penile or spongy urethra), thus containing 3 parts: prostatic, membranous, and spongy.

The process of micturition is initiated via the bladder filling, which causes the detrusor muscles to stretch. Initially, the sympathetic nerves are activated, which prevents emptying by relaxing the bladder and constricting the internal urethral sphincter. Second, the general visceral afferents from the bladder wall, due to the stretch receptors, enter the spinal cord via the pelvic splanchnic nerves (S2–S4). This signals the parasympathetic preganglionic fibers to synapse in the inferior hypogastric plexus and the postganglionic fibers to initiate bladder contraction and relaxation of the internal urethral sphincter. The general somatic efferent fibers in the pudendal nerve allow for voluntary relaxation of the external urethral sphincter, allowing the bladder to void. At the end of urination, the external urethral sphincter contracts.

Testes

The testes are the male reproductive organs responsible for the production of spermatozoa and sex hormones. They are covered by a membranous structure known as the tunica albuginea, which is located under a visceral layer called the tunica vaginalis. Their development occurs in the retroperitoneum, after which they descend into the scrotum.

The blood supply of the testes is from the testicular artery, which arises from the abdominal aorta, and the venous blood leaves through the pampiniform venous plexus. Lymphatic drainage from the testes is to the lumbar (aortic) nodes, whereas the lymph from the scrotum drains to the superficial inguinal nodes.

The **epididymis** is a convoluted duct extending from the testicle to the vas deferens. Its main purpose is to store sperm and allow for its maturation before release. The epididymis is made up of a head, body, and tail. It is in the head and body of the epididymis where the spermatozoa are stored and undergo maturation.

The **ductus deferens** enters the pelvis at the deep inguinal ring lateral to the inferior epigastric artery. As it travels, it overlaps the medial aspect of the umbilical artery and obturator neurovascular bundle. It then travels superior to the ureter posterior to the bladder and becomes dilated to be the ampulla at its terminal junction. The ductus deferens contains fructose, a nutrient source to spermatozoa. The superior hypogastric plexus (sympathetic) and the pelvic splanchnic nerves (parasympathetic) innervate the ductus deferens.

Seminal Vesicles

The **seminal vesicles** consist of lobulated glandular structures, which originate from the diverticula of the ductus deferens. They are found inferolateral to the ductus deferens ampullae. The seminal vesicles, which extend superiorly from the prostate gland between the bladder and the rectum, join the ductus deferens near their end, forming the ejaculatory ducts. The ejaculatory ducts pass through the prostate gland and open into the prostatic urethra at the seminal colliculus. The ductus deferens and the ejaculatory ducts perform peristaltic contractions of its muscular layers to push the spermatozoa with seminal fluid toward the urethra. The **seminal fluid** secreted by the seminal vesicles contributes to the quality of the semen and is rich in fructose, choline, and other proteins that provide nutrients to the spermatozoa. The ducts of the seminal vesicles join with the ductus deferens forming the ejaculatory ducts.

Prostate

The **prostate** is situated immediately inferior to the bladder, posterior to the pubic symphysis, and anterior to the rectum. It has a base at the bladder neck where the urethra exits the bladder and enters the prostate and an apex resting on the pelvic floor.

The prostate is anatomically divided into 5 lobes: the anterior, middle, posterior, and the right and left lateral lobes. Glandular tissue is the main component of the prostate, together with smooth muscle and fibrous tissue. The prostate also contributes to the semen and secretes **prostate-specific antigen**, prostaglandins, and other proteins. The secretions of the prostate add alkalinity to the ejaculate and produce the distinctive odor of semen. The prostatic ducts receive semen from the ejaculatory ducts, which empty into a groove between the urethral crest and the prostatic urethra called the prostatic sinus.

Urethral Crest

The urethral crest is found on the posterior aspect of the prostatic urethra with several openings bilaterally to receive seminal fluid from the prostatic ducts. The seminal colliculus, also referred to as verumontanum, is an enlargement of the urethral crest that serves as an opening for the ejaculatory ducts and the prostatic utricle.

Erection and Ejaculation

Erection is a process that is influenced by the parasympathetic nervous system and muscular contraction. The parasympathetic fibers from the pelvic splanchnic nerves cause arterial dilation of the erectile tissue, leading to enlargement of the corpora cavernosa and corpus spongiosum. Contraction of the bulbospongiosus and ischiocavernosus muscles allows for maintained erections. *Point* for parasympathetics (erection) and *Shoot* for **s**ympathetics (ejaculation) is a useful mnemonic to remember these associations.

Stimulation of the sympathetic fibers causes contraction of the smooth muscles of the ejaculatory tract, thus resulting in ejection of semen. **Ejaculation** is initiated by stimulation of the glans penis, which causes contractions of the bulbospongiosus muscles compressing the urethra to expel the ejaculate. Sympathetic stimulation prevents mixing of semen and urine by contracting the sphincter of the bladder.

Technique

Transabdominal (Suprapubic) Views of Abdomen/Pelvis

SUPRAPUBIC MALE PELVIS
Longitudinal (Sagittal/ Parasagittal)
FIG. 11.1

This examination is best performed when the patient's urinary bladder is full. If the urinary bladder is not at least partially full, bowel gas shadowing can interfere substantially with ultrasound (US) examination in this area. A full bladder displaces loops of bowel superiorly and provides an excellent acoustic window for US examination of pelvic structures behind the bladder.

With the patient in the supine position and properly draped, the heel of a curved array probe (nonmarker side) should be placed just over (or just above) the pubic symphysis with the marker side directed toward the head. Adjust the probe position and tilt until pelvic landmarks and structures can be identified. Urine, like all fluids, appears anechoic, and the bladder wall appears hyperechoic. In longitudinal views, full bladders are roughly triangular in shape with the apex pointing superiorly. Posterior to the bladder, identify the honeycomb appearance of seminal vesicles and the prostate. Scanning carefully across the prostate from right to left and back again, attempt to identify the urethral opening into the prostate at the bladder neck.

Figure 11.1 Normal longitudinal (sagittal/parasagittal) suprapubic view of the male pelvis.

SUPRAPUBIC MALE PELVIS
Transverse
FIG. 11.2

After completing the suprapubic examination of the pelvis in the longitudinal plane, rotate the probe 90 degrees counterclockwise so that the marker side is directed to the right and position the probe face just superior to the pubic symphysis. Adjust the probe position and tilt until pelvic landmarks and structures can be identified. In transverse views, full bladders are roughly rectangular in shape. Scanning carefully superiorly and inferiorly, identify the bladder and the hypoechoic "bow-tie" appearance of the seminal vesicles posterior to the bladder.

Rectus abdominis m.
Urinary bladder
Seminal vesicles

Rectus abdominis m.
Urinary bladder
Seminal vesicles
Rectovesical pouch
Gas shadowing from rectum

Figure 11.2 Normal transverse suprapubic view of the male pelvis.

CLINICAL APPLICATIONS

Focused Assessment with Sonography for Trauma (FAST) Examination for Detection of Intraperitoneal Bleeding

In the supine patient, free intraperitoneal fluid or large amounts of blood from the abdominal viscera typically accumulate in the following locations: hepatorenal space (Morison's pouch), splenorenal space, and in the pelvis in the pouch of Douglas in females and the retrovesical pouch in males. Chapter 12 describes the FAST examination performed to identify these spaces with examples of fluid accumulation.

Ruptured Urinary Bladder

Fractures of the pelvis or injuries at the inferior portion of the anterior abdominal wall may rupture a distended urinary bladder. Urine may escape extraperitoneally or intraperitoneally. In instances in which the rupture takes place at the superior portion of the urinary bladder, this results into extravasation of urine into the peritoneal cavity. Posterior rupture of the urinary bladder results in extravasation of urine extraperitoneally into the perineum.

Bladder Thickening

Bladder thickening is relative to the degree of urinary bladder distention. It ranges from >3 mm when distended to >5 mm when nondistended. If the bladder is well distended, then diffuse bladder wall thickening is due to urinary bladder obstruction, neurogenic bladder, and infections (cystitis). Focal urinary bladder thickening typically is due to malignancy such as transitional cell carcinoma.

Suprapubic Catheter Placement

Suprapubic catheter placement refers to the procedure in which a drainage tube is inserted into the urinary bladder under US guidance. This is because the placement of a urethral catheter is either contraindicated or unsuccessful. Typical indications for suprapubic catheter placements include urinary retention, severe benign prostatic hyperplasia, morbid obesity, urethras strictures, and trauma, among others.

12

Focused Assessment with Sonography for Trauma (FAST)

Focused assessment with sonography for trauma (FAST) is used in the setting of blunt or penetrating thoracoabdominal trauma to detect the presence of free fluid (presumed to be blood in trauma patients until proven otherwise) in the pericardial space, the pleural spaces, the right and left upper quadrants of the abdomen, and the pelvis. In the extended FAST (eFAST) examination, the lung fields are additionally examined for the presence of pneumothorax. The FAST (or eFAST) examination is noninvasive and performed at the bedside in the emergency department (ED). Patients can be continuously monitored and treated in the ED because patient transport is not required and negative or equivocal examinations can be repeated as patient hemodynamic status changes. Although organ injuries such as liver lacerations or splenic fractures can sometimes be seen during the FAST examination, it is not intended for this purpose and is not a sensitive method for detecting organ/soft tissue injury. The FAST examination is accurate and sensitive for its intended purpose, that is, detecting free fluid in the previously listed anatomical locations.

Patient Positioning

In the ED, patients presenting with thoracoabdominal trauma are commonly placed in the supine position for observation, monitoring, and treatment. **Trendelenburg position**ing (tilting the bed 15–30 degrees such that the head is lower than the feet) increases intraperitoneal fluid pooling in the upper quadrants, increasing the sensitivity of the FAST examination in these locations. Reverse Trendelenburg positioning (tilting the bed such that the feet are lower than the head) increases fluid pooling in the lower parts of the pleural spaces (**costodiaphragmatic recesses**) and in the pelvis, increasing the sensitivity of the examination in these sites.

Probe Selection

For the FAST examination, either a microconvex phased array (cardiac) probe or a curved array (abdominal) probe should be selected.

Review of the Anatomy

The anatomy and scanning techniques for the FAST examination are the same anatomy and techniques used for ultrasound (US) scanning of the heart (subxiphoid 4-chamber or parasternal long axis views), the right and left upper quadrants of the abdomen, and suprapubic views of the pelvis. The additional knowledge and skills required for the FAST examination are the ability to recognize the appearance of free fluid (anechoic) and understanding the sites where free fluid commonly accumulates relative to the main structures in each of these locations.

Right Upper Quadrant

Technique

If the patient can cooperate, the palm of the right hand should be placed behind the head, abducting the arm and helping to open up the intercostal spaces on the right. The probe should be placed along the mid-axillary line at about the horizontal level of the xiphisternal junction with the probe marker directed superiorly. The probe face should be rotated until it is parallel to the intercostal spaces (the intercostal oblique orientation), which minimizes rib shadowing over the structures of interest and brings the probe into closer alignment with the typical orientation of the right kidney. Identify the speckled appearance of the liver and the hyperechoic stripe representing the diaphragm over the curving superior surface of the liver. The probe face should be tilted

posteriorly until the interface between the visceral surface of the liver and the right kidney comes into view. The potential space at the hepatorenal recess is commonly referred to as **Morison's pouch**. This is the most dependent site in the peritoneal space above the transverse mesocolon and so is a common location for free fluid accumulation in the upper abdomen. The hepatorenal recess should be carefully and completely scanned for any anechoic fluid collections.

Next, slide the probe superiorly (1 or 2 intercostal spaces) until the superior surface of the liver, the diaphragm, and the lower part of the right hemithorax can be seen in the image. In the presence of normally aerated lung,

Figure 12.1 Upper panels: normal right upper quadrant ultrasound view including most of the hepatorenal interface. Lower panels: artist's rendering of the same view with free fluid accumulation in the potential space at the hepatorenal recess (Morison's pouch).

the hyperechoic diaphragm creates a mirror image **artifact** (a structure not normally present but visible in an image) over the lung fields such that the speckled appearance of the liver is mirrored over the right hemithorax/pleural space. The presence of free fluid in the pleural space (hemothorax or pleural effusion) abolishes the mirror image artifact, and the space above the diaphragm appears anechoic, often with atelectatic lung floating in and out of view with respiratory efforts. In addition, look carefully for any free fluid accumulation in the right subphrenic space, the potential space between the diaphragm and the superior surface of the liver.

RIGHT UPPER QUADRANT
Longitudinal (Intercostal Oblique)
FIG. 12.3

Next, slide the probe inferiorly until the inferior edge of the liver (liver tip) and inferior pole of the right kidney can be seen in the image. Free fluid may accumulate around the inferior edge of the liver before becoming visible in the potential space at the hepatorenal recess (Morison's pouch).

Figure 12.2 Upper panels: normal right upper quadrant ultrasound view including the right hemithorax, diaphragm, liver, and upper part of the hepatorenal recess. Lower panels: artist's rendering of the same view with free fluid accumulations in the right pleural and right subphrenic spaces.

Free fluid at liver edge

Liver

Kidney

Free fluid in Morison's pouch

Figure 12.3 Upper panels: normal right upper quadrant ultrasound view including the inferior edge of the liver and inferior part of the hepatorenal interface. Lower panels: artist's rendering of the same view with free fluid accumulation at the inferior edge of the liver tracking into the inferior part of Morison's pouch.

Left Upper Quadrant

Technique

LEFT UPPER QUADRANT
Longitudinal (Intercostal Oblique)
FIG. 12.4

If the patient can cooperate, the palm of the left hand should be placed behind the head, abducting the arm and helping to open up intercostal spaces on the left. The probe should be placed along the posterior axillary line 1 or 2 intercostal spaces above the level of the xiphisternal junction with the probe marker directed superiorly. Note that the left upper quadrant probe position is both more posterior and more superior than it is for the right upper quadrant views. The probe face should be rotated until it is parallel to the intercostal spaces (the intercostal oblique orientation), which minimizes rib shadowing over the spleen and left kidney. Identify the speckled appearance of the spleen and the hyperechoic stripe of the diaphragm curving over the superior surface of the spleen. Fan the probe face slightly anteriorly until the interface between the spleen and left kidney can be identified. In the left upper quadrant, free fluid most commonly accumulates in the left subphrenic space between the diaphragm and superior surface of the spleen and to a lesser extent in the potential space at the splenorenal recess. Carefully scan the left subphrenic space and splenorenal recess for any free fluid collections.

LEFT UPPER QUADRANT
Longitudinal (Intercostal Oblique)
FIG. 12.5

Next, slide the probe superiorly (1 or 2 intercostal spaces) until the spleen, the diaphragm, and the lower part of the left hemithorax can be seen in the image. In the presence of a normally aerated lung, the hyperechoic

Free fluid in left subphrenic space

Free fluid in splenorenal recess

Spleen

Kidney

Diaphragm

Figure 12.4 Upper panels: normal left upper quadrant ultrasound view including the diaphragm, spleen, and left kidney. Lower panels: artist's rendering of the same view with free fluid accumulation in the left subphrenic space and splenorenal recess.

diaphragm creates a mirror image artifact over the lung fields such that the speckled appearance of the spleen is mirrored over the left hemithorax/pleural space. The presence of free fluid in the pleural space (hemothorax or **pleural effusion**) abolishes the mirror image artifact and the space above the diaphragm appears anechoic, often with atelectatic lung floating in and out of view with respiratory efforts. In this position, look again for any free fluid accumulation between the diaphragm and the spleen (left subphrenic space).

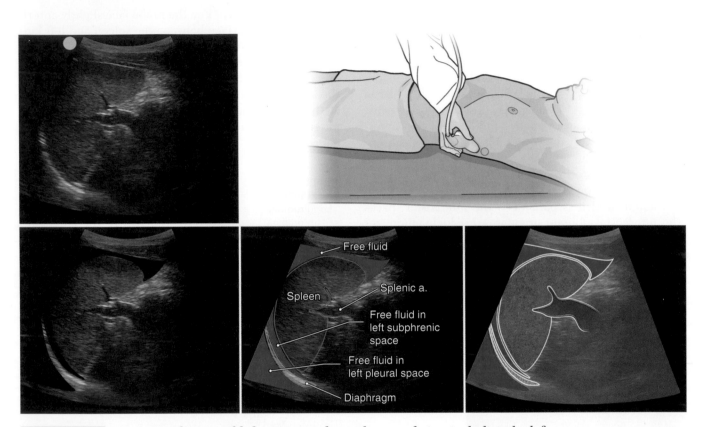

Figure 12.5 Upper panels: normal left upper quadrant ultrasound view including the left hemithorax, diaphragm, and spleen. Lower panels: artist's rendering of the same view with free fluid accumulations in the left pleural and subphrenic spaces.

Suprapubic Views of Abdomen/Pelvis

Technique

SUPRAPUBIC FEMALE PELVIS
Longitudinal (Sagittal/Parasagittal)
FIG. 12.6

At the pelvic inlet, the inferior extent of abdominal peritoneum drapes over pelvic viscera. In females, the peritoneum covers the fundus and body of the uterus and extends laterally over the uterine tubes to the pelvic walls as the broad ligaments. Peritoneum extending anteriorly from the uterus and reflecting onto the urinary bladder forms a relatively shallow space, the vesicouterine pouch, between the anterior/inferior aspect of the uterus and the urinary bladder. Peritoneum covering the posterior/superior aspect of the uterus and uterine cervix descends to just above the posterior fornix of the vagina and then reflects onto the anterior surface of the rectum forming a deep potential space, the rectouterine pouch. The rectouterine pouch is commonly referred to clinically as the **pouch of Douglas**.

The rectouterine pouch is the most dependent part of the peritoneal space in the supine position, and so US

Urinary bladder

Uterus

Free fluid in rectouterine pouch of Douglas

Figure 12.6 Upper panels: normal longitudinal (sagittal/parasagittal) suprapubic view of the female pelvis. Lower panel: artist's rendering of the same view with intraperitoneal free fluid accumulating in the rectouterine pouch of Douglas and over the fundus of the uterus toward the vesicouterine pouch.

examination in these locations is sensitive to relatively small amounts of intraperitoneal free fluid. Unfortunately, if the urinary bladder is not at least partially full, bowel gas shadowing can interfere substantially with US examination in this area. A full urinary bladder displaces loops of bowel superiorly and provides an excellent acoustic window for US examination of pelvic structures behind the urinary bladder. Because of this, at least one FAST examination should be performed along with the initial assessment of patients presenting with thoracoabdominal trauma before placing a Foley catheter.

The heel of the probe (nonmarker side) should be placed just over (or just above) the pubic symphysis with the marker side directed toward the head. Adjust the probe position and tilt until pelvic landmarks and structures can be identified. Urine, like all fluids, appears anechoic and the urinary bladder wall appears hyperechoic. In longitudinal views, full urinary bladders are roughly triangular in shape with the apex pointing superiorly.

Posterior to the urinary bladder, identify the fundus and body of the uterus, the hyperechoic endometrial stripe, and the cervix. Scan carefully to the left and right of the midline looking for any free fluid collections in the rectouterine and vesicouterine pouches.

SUPRAPUBIC MALE PELVIS
Longitudinal (Sagittal/Parasagittal)
FIG. 12.7

At the pelvic inlet, the inferior extent of abdominal peritoneum drapes over pelvic viscera. In males, peritoneum draping over the urinary bladder reflects onto the anterior surface of the rectum, forming the rectovesical pouch. The superior poles of the seminal vesicles are just beneath the inferior extent of the rectovesical pouch.

The heel of the probe (nonmarker side) should be placed just over (or just above) the pubic symphysis with the marker side directed toward the head. Adjust the probe position and tilt until pelvic landmarks and structures can be identified. Identify the urinary bladder, the seminal vesicles and the prostate gland. Scan carefully along the superior/posterior aspect of the urinary bladder for any free fluid collection in the rectovesical pouch.

Figure 12.7 Upper panels: normal longitudinal (sagittal/parasagittal) suprapubic view of the male pelvis. Lower panel: artist's rendering of the same view with intraperitoneal free fluid accumulating in the rectovesical pouch.

SUPRAPUBIC FEMALE PELVIS
Transverse
FIG. 12.8

After completing the suprapubic examination of the pelvis in the longitudinal plane, rotate the probe 90 degrees counterclockwise so that the marker side is directed to the right and position the probe face just superior to the pubic symphysis. Adjust the probe position and tilt until pelvic landmarks and structures can be identified. In transverse views, full urinary bladders are roughly rectangular in shape.

Identify the urinary bladder, uterus, and endometrial stripe. Scan carefully superiorly and inferiorly along the uterus, looking for any free fluid collections in the rectouterine and/or vesicouterine pouches.

SUPRAPUBIC MALE PELVIS
Transverse
FIG. 12.9

After completing the suprapubic examination of the pelvis in the longitudinal plane, rotate the probe 90 degrees counterclockwise so that the marker side is directed to the right and position the probe face just superior to the pubic symphysis. Adjust the probe position and tilt until pelvic landmarks and structures can be identified. In transverse views, full urinary bladders are roughly rectangular in shape.

Identify the urinary bladder and the seminal vesicles. Scan carefully along the superior/posterior aspect of the urinary bladder just superior to the seminal vesicles for any free fluid collection in the rectovesical pouch.

Figure 12.8 Upper panels: normal transverse suprapubic view of the female pelvis. Lower panel: artist's rendering of the same view with intraperitoneal free fluid accumulating in the rectouterine pouch of Douglas and the vesicouterine pouch.

Figure 12.9 Upper panels: normal transverse suprapubic view of the male pelvis. Lower panel: artist's rendering of the same view with intraperitoneal free fluid accumulating in the rectovesical pouch.

Heart and Pericardial Space

SUBXIPHOID 4-CHAMBER VIEW FIG. 12.10

The **subxiphoid 4-chamber view** uses the liver as a sonographic window to view the heart and pericardium. If the patient can cooperate, flexing the knees to 90 degrees and placing the soles of the feet on the bed relaxes the abdominal musculature. To obtain this view, place the probe face just to the right of the midline 2 to 4 cm below the xiphoid process, depending on the width of the subcostal arch. The probe should be far enough below the xiphoid process so that the sides of the probe face are not pressing against ribs/costal cartilages. Next, exert pressure directly posteriorly, and then with a scooping motion, flatten the probe against the abdominal wall, directing the US beam upward and slightly toward the left shoulder. Adjust probe position and tilt until the liver, heart chambers, and **pericardium** can be identified. If needed, increase the depth setting until the posterior pericardium adjacent to the free wall of the left ventricle can

be clearly seen in the far field. If possible, ask the patient to take a deep breath, which brings the heart closer to the probe and improves image quality. Carefully scan along the heart and pericardium, looking for any free fluid or blood accumulating between the speckled-appearing myocardium and the hyperechoic pericardium.

Note: When a **microconvex phased array (cardiac) probe** is used, many US units automatically place the screen marker dot to the right of the screen image rather than to the left of the screen image as in all other applications. If the screen marker dot is on the left of the image as usual (as it should be when a curved array or abdominal probe is used), then the marker side of the probe should be directed toward the patient's right axilla to obtain display images as shown in Figure 12.10. If the marker dot is on the right of the screen image, then the marker side of the probe should be directed toward the patient's left flank to obtain the same image orientation on the display.

Figure 12.10 Upper panels: normal subxiphoid 4-chamber view of the heart and pericardium. Lower panels: artist's rendering of the same view with free fluid in the pericardial space.

PARASTERNAL LONG AXIS VIEW
FIG. 12.11

To obtain the parasternal long axis view, place the probe face just to the left of the sternum in the third, fourth, or fifth intercostal space approximately along a line connecting the right shoulder and left nipple. This orients the probe/US beam along the long axis of the left ventricle. Adjust probe position up or down 1 intercostal space at a time as needed, until an image of the heart as shown in Figure 12.11 can be best seen. The posterior free wall of the left ventricle and adjacent posterior pericardium should be identified in the far field. The left atrium, mitral valve, inflow tract of the left ventricle, outflow tract of the left ventricle, aortic valve, and ascending aorta should be identified. The interventricular septum and outflow tract of the right ventricle should be seen in the near field. The descending thoracic aorta can often be seen just posterior to the left atrium near the position of the mitral valve annulus. The apex of the left ventricle should be beyond the edge of the display image to the left. Carefully scan along the heart and pericardium looking for any free fluid accumulating between the speckled-appearing myocardium of the left ventricle and the hyperechoic pericardium and continuing around the apex of the left ventricle and between the free wall of the right ventricle and the anterior pericardium.

Note: When a microconvex phased array (cardiac) probe is used, many US units automatically place the screen marker dot to the right of the screen image, rather than to the left of the screen image as in all other applications. If the screen marker dot is on the left of the image as usual (as it should be when a curved array or abdominal probe is used), then the marker side of the probe should be directed toward the patient's left flank to obtain display images as shown in Figure 12.11. If the marker dot is on the right of the screen image, then the marker side of the probe should be directed toward the patient's right shoulder to obtain the same image orientation on the display.

Right ventricle
Left ventricle
Mitral leaflets
Left atrium
Hemopericardium
Pericardium
Lung
Descending aorta

Figure 12.11 Upper panels: normal parasternal long axis view of the heart and pericardium. Lower panels: artist's rendering of the same view with free fluid in the pericardial space.

Multiple-Choice Questions

3 Back

1. A 50-year-old woman is brought to the emergency department because of a 5-day history of high fever and headaches. She is HIV positive, and a fungal meningitis is suspected. She undergoes an ultrasound-guided lumbar puncture. Which of the following structures or spaces will be penetrated/traversed just before the needle enters the lumbar cistern?

   a) Arachnoid mater
   b) Dura mater
   c) Epidural space
   d) Ligamentum flavum
   e) Posterior longitudinal ligament

2. A 29-year-old woman is undergoing an ultrasound-guided placement of a catheter for epidural anesthesia during labor. Which of the following structures will be penetrated just before the catheter enters the epidural space?

   a) Anterior longitudinal ligament
   b) Interspinous ligament
   c) Ligamentum flavum
   d) Multifidus muscle
   e) Thoracolumbar fascia

4 Upper Limb

1. A 27-year-old cricket bowler is undergoing an ultrasound-guided interscalene brachial plexus block before surgical repair of his radial collateral ligament of the elbow. This patient will most likely require additional regional anesthesia at another site if the surgical field

must be expanded to encroach which of the following structures?

   a) Anular ligament
   b) Lateral epicondyle of the humerus
   c) Origin of brachioradialis muscle
   d) Supinator muscle
   e) Ulnar collateral ligament

2. Following a motor vehicle collision that resulted in a comminuted fracture of the right clavicle, a 25-year-old man has developed extensive weakness/paralysis in his right upper limb. Physical examination shows weakness of both abduction and adduction of the arm, extension of the elbow, and extension of the wrist and digits. There is decreased sensation over the shoulder, posterior and lateral aspects of the arm, posterior aspect of the forearm, and dorsum of the hand laterally. An ultrasound examination of the axilla will most likely show posttraumatic changes in which of the following components of the brachial plexus?

   a) Upper trunk
   b) Lower trunk
   c) Lateral cord
   d) Posterior cord
   e) Medial cord

3. A 20-year-old college tennis player comes to the physician because of a 6-month history of progressive shoulder pain, especially while serving. Physical examination shows that flexion of the shoulder to 90 degrees accompanied by internal rotation results in severe pain under her acromion process. An ultrasound examination of her shoulder will most likely show injury of which of the following tendons?

259

a) Biceps brachii, long head
b) Infraspinatus
c) Subscapularis
d) Supraspinatus
e) Teres minor

4. A 60-year-old woman comes to the physician because of a deep aching pain in the anterior part of her shoulder for the past several weeks. Physical examination shows tenderness to palpation over her anterior shoulder, and the pain is reproduced by supination of the forearm against resistance and by flexion of the shoulder against resistance with the forearm extended and supinated. An ultrasound examination of the shoulder is most likely to show inflammatory changes in which of the following tendons?

a) Biceps brachii, long head
b) Infraspinatus
c) Subscapularis
d) Supraspinatus
e) Teres minor

5. A 78-year-old woman with end-stage renal disease and a left brachial artery/basilic vein arteriovenous fistula is admitted to the hospital because of a 2-month history of pain in her upper limb. Physical examination shows numbness and tingling in her palm and palmar aspect of the thumb and index and middle fingers of her left hand. An ultrasound examination shows an aneurysm of the brachial artery in the distal third of the arm. Which of the following muscles is most likely to exhibit weakness?

a) Adductor pollicis
b) Brachialis
c) Extensor carpi ulnaris
d) Flexor carpi ulnaris
e) Pronator teres

6. An 82-year-old woman is admitted to the emergency department because of severe pain in her right upper limb after falling forward onto her hands and knees, while rising from a chair. An x-ray of her arm shows an oblique fracture at the mid-shaft of her right humerus. Immediately after closed reduction of the fracture, she developed numbness and tingling in the limb. An ultrasound examination would most likely show injury to which of the following nerves?

a) Deep radial nerve
b) Posterior cutaneous nerve of the forearm
c) Posterior interosseous nerve
d) Radial nerve
e) Superficial radial nerve

7. Following a bar fight, a 26-year-old man is brought to the emergency department with multiple defensive stab wounds along the anterior surface of the left forearm and medial surface of the elbow and arm. An ultrasound examination shows a hematoma a few centimeters below the elbow between the flexor digitorum superficialis and flexor digitorum profundus muscles. Which of the following nerves is most likely to be affected by a hematoma in this location?

a) Deep radial nerve
b) Medial cutaneous nerve of the forearm
c) Median nerve
d) Superficial radial nerve
e) Ulnar nerve

8. A 45-year-old man comes to the physician because of a 5-week history of numbness and tingling in the ring and little fingers of his right hand. He is now concerned that he seems to be losing strength in the hand. Physical examination shows altered sensation in the palmar aspect of the ring and little fingers on the right, along with weakness of adduction of all of the digits of his right hand. Strength for flexion at the proximal and distal interphalangeal joints of all fingers is normal and equal bilaterally. An ultrasound examination shows a compression of the ulnar nerve. In which of the following locations is the compression most likely taking place?

a) Cubital tunnel
b) Supinator muscle
c) Between the heads of pronator teres muscle
d) Guyon's canal
e) Carpal tunnel

9. A 23-year old woman comes to the physician because of a 1-month history of numbness and tingling over the lateral side of the wrist, thumb, and dorsum of her hand. A month ago, she underwent a fixator pin placement for a complicated fracture of the distal radius. Physical examination shows no loss of motor function in the wrist or hand. An ultrasound examination shows a nerve entrapment. Which of the following nerves is most likely entrapped?

a) Anterior interosseous nerve
b) Dorsal cutaneous branch of the ulnar nerve
c) Posterior cutaneous nerve of the forearm
d) Posterior interosseous nerve
e) Superficial radial nerve

5 Lower Limb

1. A 75-year-old woman comes to the physician because of a 6-month history of cold and pale right foot. Physical examination shows a cyanotic painful cold foot. An ultrasound Doppler examination shows a thrombotic occlusion of her popliteal artery and minimal flow at the posterior tibial artery. Physical examination will most likely show absence of the pulse on which of the following locations?

   a) Lateral to the abductor hallucis
   b) Posteroinferior to the medial femoral condyle
   c) Midway between the lateral malleolus and the calcaneus
   d) Midway between the medial malleolus and the calcaneus
   e) Between the two heads of the gastrocnemius

2. An 80-year-old woman comes to the physician because of a 6-month history of progressive difficulty walking. An ultrasound Doppler examination shows occlusion of her femoral artery at the proximal part of the adductor canal and well-established collateral circulation. Which of the following arteries will most likely be responsible for the collateral circulation?

   a) Descending branch of the lateral circumflex femoral
   b) Descending genicular
   c) Medial circumflex femoral
   d) First perforating branch of deep femoral
   e) Obturator artery

3. An 85-year-old man comes to the physician because of a 6-month history of progressive difficulty walking. He was diagnosed with osteoarthritis 25 years ago. Physical examination shows pain and tightness posteriorly to his right knee. An ultrasound examination shows a large cyst in the popliteal fossa compressing the adjacent nerve descending the fossa vertically. Which of the following movement will most likely be impaired during physical examination?

   a) Dorsiflexion of the foot
   b) Flexion of the thigh
   c) Extension of the digits
   d) Extension of the leg
   e) Plantar flexion of the foot

6 Thorax: Chest Wall and Pleura

1. A 19-year-old man is brought to the emergency department 35 minutes after being involved in a motor vehicle collision. Physical examination shows swelling, inflammation, and deformation of the chest wall caused upon impact with the steering wheel during the collision. A chest x-ray shows a fracture of the sternum at the manubriosternal joint. Which of the following ribs would most likely be involved in such an injury?

   a) First
   b) Second
   c) Third
   d) Fourth
   e) Fifth

2. A 19-year-old man is brought to the emergency department 35 minutes after being involved in a motor vehicle collision. Physical examination shows a wound in the neck just above the middle of the right clavicle and first rib. A chest x-ray shows collapse of the right lung and a tension pneumothorax. Injury to which of the following structures resulted in the pneumothorax?

   a) Costal pleura
   b) Mediastinal parietal pleura
   c) Diaphragmatic parietal pleura
   d) Cupula
   e) Endothoracic fascia

3. A 19-year-old man is brought to the emergency department 35 minutes after being involved in a motor vehicle collision. Physical examination shows a wound in the neck just above the middle of the right clavicle and first rib. A chest x-ray shows collapse of the right lung and a tension pneumothorax. A chest tube is inserted and adequate local anesthesia of the chest wall before insertion of a chest tube is administered. Of the following layers, which is the deepest that must be infiltrated with the local anesthetic to achieve adequate anesthesia?

   a) Parietal pleura
   b) Visceral pleura
   c) Endothoracic fascia
   d) Intercostal muscles
   e) Subcutaneous fat

4. A 19-year-old man is brought to the emergency department 35 minutes after being involved in a motor vehicle collision. Physical examination shows a wound in the neck just above the middle of the right clavicle and first rib. A chest x-ray shows collapse of the right lung and a tension pneumothorax. A chest tube is inserted, and adequate local anesthesia of the chest wall before insertion of a chest tube is administered. Between which layers will the chest tube have to be placed to relieve the pneumothorax?

a) Between the mediastinal pleura and fibrous pericardium
b) Between the visceral and parietal layers of the pericardium
c) Between the serous and fibrous layers of the pericardium
d) Between the endothoracic fascia and parietal pleura
e) Between the parietal and visceral layers of the pleura

5. A 55-year-old woman is brought to the emergency department because of a 2-day history of sharp and localized pain over the thoracic wall during coughing. A chest x-ray shows pleural effusion. A chest tube is inserted to drain the effusion through an intercostal space. At which of the following locations is the chest tube most likely to be inserted?

a) Between the internal and external intercostal muscles
b) Inferior to the lower border of the rib
c) Superior to the upper border of the rib
d) At the middle of the intercostal space
e) Between the intercostal muscles and the posterior intercostal membrane

7 Heart

1. A 72-year-old man is admitted to the emergency department because of symptoms and signs of congestive heart failure. A transesophageal echocardiography is performed, and the ultrasound transducer is placed through the mouth to his esophagus to lie directly posteriorly to the heart. Placing the transducer in this position which of the following cardiac valves will be best visualized?

a) Valve of the inferior vena cava
b) Tricuspid
c) Pulmonary
d) Mitral
e) Aortic

2. A 65-year-old man is brought to the emergency department 30 minutes after he had an episode of intense chest pain. He describes the pain as retrosternal, radiating to the left side of his neck and shoulder and down to the medial aspect of his left arm. There is no family history of heart disease. His temperature is 98.6°F (37°C), pulse is 100/min, respirations are 22/min, and blood pressure is 130/80 mm Hg. Physical examination also shows a slight rhythmic pulsation on the chest wall

at the left fifth intercostal space is noted in the midclavicular line. Which of the following structures is most likely responsible for this pulsation?

a) Aortic arch
b) Mitral valve
c) Right atrium
d) Left atrium
e) Apex of the heart

3. A 60-year-old man is brought to the emergency department with his wife because of a 3-week history of progressively worsening difficulty breathing. He has no prior history of hospitalizations or any major illness. Physical examination shows moderate respiratory distress. An ultrasound examination of his heart shows severe aortic valve prolapse. Auscultation of this valve is best performed at which of the following locations?

a) Directly over the middle of the manubrium
b) Left fifth intercostal space, just below the nipple
c) Right lower part of the body of the sternum
d) Right second intercostal space near the lateral border of the sternum
e) Left second intercostal space near the lateral border of the sternum

4. A 65-year-old man is brought to the emergency department 30 minutes after he had an episode of intense chest pain. He describes the pain as retrosternal, radiating to the left side of his neck and shoulder and down to the medial aspect of his left arm. There is no family history of heart disease. His temperature is 98.6°F (37°C), pulse is 100/min, respirations are 22/min, and blood pressure is 130/80 mm Hg. Electrocardiography shows myocardial infarction of the anterior right ventricular wall. Which of the following arteries is most likely to be occluded?

a) Anterior interventricular artery
b) Posterior interventricular artery
c) Circumflex
d) Acute marginal branch of the right coronary artery
e) Artery of the conus

5. A 42-year-old woman is brought to the emergency department because of a 2-day history of severe chest pain, dyspnea, tachycardia, cough, and fever. An ultrasound examination shows pericardial effusion, and a pericardiocentesis is performed via the infrasternal angle. The patient is agitated and constantly moves. The needle pierces the visceral pericardium and enters the heart. Which of the following cardiac chambers would be the first to be penetrated by the needle?

a) Right ventricle
b) Left ventricle
c) Right atrium
d) Left atrium
e) The left cardiac apex

a) The hepatopancreatic ampulla
b) The cystic duct
c) The common bile duct
d) The left hepatic duct
e) The infundibulum of the gallbladder

8 Abdomen

1. A 70-year-old man is brought to the emergency department because of a 2-hour history of severe pain radiating from his lower back toward his pubic symphysis. Ultrasound examination shows a kidney stone obstructing his right ureter. At which of the following locations is the stone most likely lodged?

   a) Major calyx
   b) Minor calyx
   c) Pelvic brim
   d) Midportion of the ureter
   e) Between the pelvic brim and the urinary bladder

2. A 70-year-old man is brought to the emergency department because of a 2-hour history of severe pain radiating from his lower back toward his pubic symphysis. Ultrasound examination shows a kidney stone obstructing his right ureter. Which of the following nerves is most likely responsible for conducting the sensation of pain?

   a) Lateral femoral cutaneous
   b) Ilioinguinal
   c) Obturator
   d) Subcostal
   e) Iliohypogastric

3. A 45-year-old man is brought to the emergency department because of a 2-day history of abdominal pain, vomiting, and fever. The pain started as poorly localized to the epigastrium but became progressively sharp in nature and radiated to the right hypochondriac region. The pain now radiates to the right shoulder. Physical examination shows yellowing of the sclerae, soft and tender abdomen, and a positive Murphy's sign. An ultrasound examination of his abdomen shows thickened gallbladder, with several echogenic gallstones and dilation of the biliary tree. Laboratory studies show elevated serum bilirubin, alanine aminotransferase (ALT), aspartate aminotransferase (AST), alkaline phosphatase (ALP), and gamma-glutamyl transferase (GGT) and increased prothrombin time. Endoscopic retrograde cholangiopancreatography shows an obstruction along the extrahepatic biliary tree with normal pancreatic duct flow. Which of the structures is most likely obstructed?

4. A 45-year-old man is brought to the emergency department because of a 2-day history of abdominal pain, vomiting, and fever. The pain started as poorly localized to the epigastrium but became progressively sharp in nature and radiated to the right hypochondriac region. The pain now radiates to the right shoulder. Physical examination shows yellowing of the sclerae, soft and tender abdomen, and a positive Murphy's sign. An ultrasound examination of his abdomen shows thickened gallbladder, with several echogenic gallstones and dilation of the biliary tree. Laboratory studies show elevated serum bilirubin, alanine aminotransferase (ALT), aspartate aminotransferase (AST), alkaline phosphatase (ALP), and gamma-glutamyl transferase (GGT) and increased prothrombin time. A laparoscopic cholecystectomy is performed using the triangle of Calot as landmark. Which of the following are the boundaries of the triangle of Calot?

   a) Cystic artery, common hepatic duct, bile duct
   b) Gallbladder, hepatic duct, bile duct
   c) Inferior border of the liver, cystic duct, common hepatic duct
   d) Inferior border of liver, bile duct, common hepatic duct
   e) Cystic artery, inferior border of liver, bile duct

5. A 45-year-old man is brought to the emergency department because of a 2-day history of abdominal pain, vomiting, and fever. The pain started as poorly localized to the epigastrium but became progressively sharp in nature and radiated to the right hypochondriac region. The pain now radiates to the right shoulder. Physical examination shows yellowing of the sclerae, soft and tender abdomen, and a positive Murphy's sign. An ultrasound examination of his abdomen shows thickened gallbladder, with several echogenic gallstones and dilation of the biliary tree. Laboratory studies show elevated serum bilirubin, alanine aminotransferase (ALT), aspartate aminotransferase (AST), alkaline phosphatase (ALP), and gamma-glutamyl transferase (GGT) and increased prothrombin time. A laparoscopic cholecystectomy is performed using the triangle of Calot as landmark. Which of the following structures would most likely be identified and ligated within the triangle?

a) Cystic artery
b) Right hepatic artery
c) Bile duct
d) Cystic duct
e) Right hepatic duct

6. A 45-year-old man is brought to the emergency department because of a 2-day history of abdominal pain, vomiting, and fever. The pain started as poorly localized to the epigastrium but became progressively sharp in nature and radiated to the right hypochondriac region. The pain now radiates to the right shoulder. Physical examination shows yellowing of the sclerae, soft and tender abdomen, and a positive Murphy's sign. An ultrasound examination of his abdomen shows thickened gallbladder, with several echogenic gallstones and dilation of the biliary tree. Laboratory studies show elevated serum bilirubin, alanine aminotransferase (ALT), aspartate aminotransferase (AST), alkaline phosphatase (ALP), and gamma-glutamyl transferase (GGT) and increased prothrombin time. A laparoscopic cholecystectomy is performed using the triangle of Calot as landmark. During laparoscopic cholecystectomy the scope is passed into the greater sac through a small port in the anterior abdominal wall. Which organ is the surgeon unable to view directly?

a) Ileum
b) Jejunum
c) Pancreas
d) Stomach
e) Transverse colon

 ## 9 Neck, Face, Eye

1. A 55-year-old woman comes to the physician because of a 6-month history of progressive swelling on the left side of her face. Physical examination shows a painless swelling over the parotid gland, and an ultrasound-guided needle biopsy shows a malignant parotid tumor. A parotidectomy is performed. Postoperatively, physical examination shows weakness at the inferior portion of the orbicularis oris. Which of the following nerves was most likely injured?

a) Mandibular division of the trigeminal
b) Marginal mandibular branch of facial
c) Zygomatic branch of facial
d) Buccal branch of facial
e) Buccal nerve

2. A 45-year-old woman comes to the physician because of a 6-month history of progressive swelling of the anterior portion of her neck. Physical examination shows an

enlarged thyroid gland. An ultrasound-guided needle biopsy of the thyroid gland shows a benign tumor measuring 3 × 6 cm. A partial thyroidectomy is performed. Postoperatively, physical examination shows hoarseness and difficulty breathing on exertion. Which of the following nerves was most likely injured during the thyroidectomy?

a) Internal branch of superior laryngeal
b) External branch of superior laryngeal
c) Recurrent laryngeal
d) Ansa cervicalis
e) Vagus

3. A 68-year-old man is brought to the emergency department because of a 2-day history of feeling dizzy and falling. His pulse is 110/min, blood pressure is 190/110 mm Hg, and respirations are 21/min. Physical examination shows carotid bruits bilaterally. An ultrasound Doppler examination shows 90% occlusion in both common carotid arteries proximal to their division into external and internal carotid arteries. A stent is placed in both common carotid arteries, and the flow is restored bilaterally. Postoperatively, physical examination shows that his tongue is deviated to the right when he is asked to protrude it. Which of the following nerves was most likely injured during the procedure?

a) Right lingual
b) Right hypoglossal
c) Left hypoglossal
d) Right glossopharyngeal
e) Right vagus

4. A 59-year-old man was brought to the emergency department after falling from a 3-story scaffolding. On arrival, the patient is unconscious with a fractured jaw, broken teeth, facial lacerations, an open tibial fracture and on hypovolemic shock. An emergency central venous line is inserted to the internal jugular vein. Which of the following is a reliable landmark to access this vein?

a) The interval between the sternal and clavicular heads of the sternocleidomastoid muscle
b) The lateral border of sternocleidomastoid muscle
c) Midclavicular line
d) Parasternal line
e) Jugular notch

5. A 45-year-old woman comes to the physician because of a 6-month history of progressive swelling of the anterior portion of her neck. Physical examination shows an enlarged thyroid gland. An ultrasound-guided needle biopsy of the thyroid gland shows a benign tumor

measuring 3 × 6 cm. A partial thyroidectomy is performed. Postoperatively, physical examination shows hoarseness and difficulty breathing on exertion. Which of the following vessels accompany the nerve injured during the thyroidectomy procedure?

a) Inferior thyroid artery
b) Inferior and superior thyroid arteries
c) Superior thyroid artery and vein
d) Superior and middle thyroid veins
e) Superior, middle, and inferior thyroid veins

6. A 55-year-old man is brought to the emergency department 45 minutes after being involved in a motor vehicle collision. He is in hypovolemic shock. Physical examination shows an unconscious man with multiple lacerations on his face and blood within the oral cavity. An emergency airway is established with a cricothyroidotomy, and a central venous line is inserted in the subclavian vein via a supraclavicular approach. An artery is injured during the cricothyroidotomy procedure, causing a delay in establishing the airway. Which of the following arteries was most likely injured?

a) Inferior thyroid
b) A branch from the costocervical trunk
c) Transverse cervical
d) Cricothyroid
e) Superior laryngeal

7. A 40-year-old man comes to the emergency department because of a 2-month history of a progressive swelling on the right side of his face underneath the mandible. Physical examination shows a hard, nontender mass in the right submandibular region. An ultrasound-guided biopsy of the mass shows a mucoepidermoid carcinoma of the submandibular gland. A submandibulectomy is performed removing the gland and its duct. Which of the following nerves need to be identified and preserved during the procedure?

a) Nerve to mylohyoid
b) Lingual
c) Inferior alveolar
d) Buccal
e) Glossopharyngeal

⑩ Female Pelvis

1. A 55-year-old woman is brought to the emergency department because of an enlarged and painful abdomen. She has chronic renal failure for the past 3 years. An ultrasound examination shows ascites in the peritoneal cavity. An ultrasound-guided needle is placed through the posterior vaginal fornix to drain the fluid. Which of the following spaces/pouches will the needle enter to drain the fluid?

a) Uterovesical pouch
b) Pararectal space
c) Paravesical space
d) Rectouterine pouch
e) Superficial perineal pouch

2. A 38-year-old woman is admitted to the hospital for a scheduled tubal ligation. Two days after the procedure she has high fever and shows symptoms of hypovolemic shock. An ultrasound examination of her pelvis shows a large hematoma adjacent to the external iliac artery. Which of the following arteries is most likely injured during this procedure?

a) Ovarian
b) Ascending branch of uterine
c) Descending branch of uterine
d) Superior vesical
e) Inferior vesical

3. A 39-year-old woman undergoes bilateral oophorectomy with ligation of the ovarian vessels. Three years ago, she had a prophylactic bilateral mastectomy because of a recent BRCA1 diagnosis. Both her mother and older sister have been diagnosed with breast cancer. Which of the following structures is most likely at risk of injury when the ovarian vessels are ligated?

a) Uterine artery
b) Pudendal nerve
c) Internal pudendal artery
d) Vaginal artery
e) Ureter

4. A 42-year-old woman comes to the physician because of a 6-month history of heavy painful menstrual bleedings. She has extremely heavy periods and abdominal pain, which has resulted in anemia. An ultrasound examination shows several large uterine leiomyomas. A hysterectomy is performed, and the uterine artery is identified and ligated. Which of the following adjacent structures is most susceptible to iatrogenic injury during ligation of this artery?

a) Obturator nerve
b) Internal iliac artery
c) Lumbosacral trunk
d) Ureter
e) Internal iliac vein

11 Male Pelvis

1. A 25-year-old man comes to the physician because of a 2-month history of a painless, swelling in his right scrotum. Physical examination shows a nontender, palpable mass on the right testis. An ultrasound examination of the right scrotum shows a 3 × 3 cm intratesticular mass. A radical orchiectomy is performed. Biopsy of the mass shows testicular seminoma. Which of the following lymph nodes will most likely receive metastatic cells first?

   a) External iliac
   b) Superficial inguinal
   c) Deep inguinal
   d) Internal iliac
   e) Lumbar

2. A 24-year-woman is brought to the emergency department with a report of having been sexually assaulted 24 hours earlier. She says that a man she had met at a campus party walked her to her apartment, where he assaulted and raped her, including vaginal penetration. She did not report the assault to the police but confided in a friend, who encouraged her to seek medical care. In collecting samples of an evidence-collection kit, two sterile dry cotton-tipped swabs are used simultaneously to collect sample. Fluids from her vagina are collected for DNA and fructose examination. Which of the following organs is most likely responsible for fructose production?

   a) Kidneys
   b) Prostate gland
   c) Testis
   d) Seminal vesicles
   e) Bulbourethral (Cowper) glands

3. A 75-year-old man comes to the physician because of a 6-month history of progressive dysuria, nocturia, and urinary urgency. Laboratory studies show high levels of prostate-specific antigen, and transurethral biopsy shows prostate cancer. A radical prostatectomy is performed. Postoperatively, he experiences urinary incontinence secondary to paralysis of the external urethral sphincter. Which of the following nerves was most likely injured during the operation?

   a) Parasympathetic preganglionic
   b) Pelvic splanchnic (S2–S4)
   c) General somatic efferent from pudendal
   d) Sympathetic fibers from superior hypogastric plexus
   e) General visceral afferent

12 Focused Assessment With Sonography for Trauma (FAST)

1. A 63-year-old woman is brought to the emergency department because of a fall from a 3-m (10-ft)-high balcony of her apartment. She has severe chest pain, dyspnea, tachypnea, tachycardia, and cough. A radiograph of the hips and lower limb shows multiple spiral fractures. After 2 hours she develops signs of Beck's triad. Which of the following ultrasound views will most likely identify fluid in the pericardial cavity?

   a) Parasternal long axis
   b) Parasternal short axis
   c) Apical
   d) Subcostal inferior vena cava

2. A 55-year-old woman is brought to the emergency department because of a 1-week history of progressive pain in the right side of her lower abdomen. She experienced a feeling of abdominal fullness and discomfort. She also cannot lie down easily. A focused assessment with sonography for trauma (FAST) examination and a computed tomography scan of the abdomen are performed. A diagnosis of an ovarian tumor is made. Which of the following ultrasound views will most likely identify fluid in the abdominal cavity in this patient?

   a) Hepatorenal
   b) Left subphrenic
   c) Left splenorenal
   d) Longitudinal suprapubic
   e) Suprapubic transverse

3. A 55-year-old man is brought to the emergency department 45 minutes after being involved in a motor vehicle collision. Physical examination shows a wound in the neck just above the middle of the right clavicle in the first rib. A radiograph of the thorax shows collapse of the right lung and a tension pneumothorax. Which of the following is the typical ultrasonographic finding for the diagnosis of pneumothorax?

   a) Absence of pleural sliding
   b) Presence of A lines
   c) Presence of B lines
   d) Presence of E lines
   e) Presence of lung pulse

4. A 35-year-old woman is admitted to the emergency department 45 minutes after being involved in a motor vehicle collision. Physical examination shows that her left lower back is bruised and swollen. She has a sharp pain during respiration. A radiograph of her chest shows a fracture of the 11th rib on the left side. Which of the following organs would most likely sustain an injury?

   a) Kidney
   b) Pancreas
   c) Lung
   d) Spleen
   e) Liver

5. A 75-year-old woman is brought to the emergency department because of a 2-hour history of severe chest pain, dyspnea, tachycardia, cough, and fever. An ultrasound examination shows significant pericardial effusion. A pericardiocentesis is performed, and the needle is inserted using the subxiphoid approach. The needle passes too deeply, piercing the visceral pericardium and enters the heart. Which of the following chambers would be the first to be penetrated by the needle?

   a) Left ventricle
   b) Left cardiac apex
   c) Right atrium
   d) Right ventricle
   e) Left atrium

6. A 28-year-old woman is brought to the emergency department because of a 3-hour history of sharp pain in the left lower quadrant. An ultrasound examination shows a ruptured ectopic pregnancy close to the left ovary. There is a small amount of fluid in the abdominal cavity from the bleeding from the rupture site. Which of the following locations is the fluid most likely present?

   a) Rectouterine pouch (of Douglas)
   b) Hepatorenal pouch (of Morison)
   c) Vesicouterine pouch
   d) Right subphrenic space
   e) Paracolic gutters

Answers

Chapter 3

1. a) Arachnoid mater
2. c) Ligamentum flavum

Chapter 4

1. e) Ulnar collateral ligament
2. d) Posterior cord
3. d) Supraspinatus
4. a) Biceps brachii, long head
5. e) Pronator teres
6. d) Radial nerve
7. c) Median nerve
8. d) Guyon's canal
9. e) Superficial radial nerve

Chapter 5

1. d) Midway between the medial malleolus and the calcaneus
2. a) Descending branch of the lateral circumflex femoral
3. e) Plantar flexion of the foot

Chapter 6

1. b) Second
2. d) Cupula
3. a) Parietal pleura
4. e) Between the parietal and visceral layers of the pleura
5. c) Superior to the upper border of the rib

Chapter 7

1. d) Mitral
2. e) Apex of the heart
3. d) Right second intercostal space near the lateral border of the sternum
4. e) Artery of the conus
5. a) Right ventricle

Chapter 8

1. c) Pelvic brim
2. b) Ilioinguinal
3. c) The common bile duct
4. c) Inferior border of the liver, cystic duct, common hepatic duct
5. a) Cystic artery
6. c) Pancreas

Chapter 9

1. b) Marginal mandibular branch of facial
2. c) Recurrent laryngeal
3. b) Right hypoglossal
4. a) The interval between the sternal and clavicular heads of the sternocleidomastoid muscle
5. a) Inferior thyroid artery
6. d) Cricothyroid
7. b) Lingual

Chapter 10

1. d) Rectouterine pouch
2. a) Ovarian arteries
3. e) Ureter
4. d) Ureter

Chapter 11

1. e) Lumbar
2. d) Seminal vesicles
3. c) General somatic efferent from pudendal

Chapter 12

1. a) Parasternal long axis
2. a) Hepatorenal
3. a) Absence of pleural sliding
4. d) Spleen
5. d) Right ventricle
6. a) Rectouterine pouch (of Douglas)

Index

Note: Page numbers followed by "f" indicate figures, "t" indicate tables and "b" indicate boxes.

Index

Index

Index